INTERROGATING INCEST

Interrogating Incest explores the relationship between feminism and the work of Michel Foucault around the specific topic of incest. Whereas sociologists initially concerned themselves with the origins and function of the taboo, later questions have stemmed from feminist work in this area. These have often theorised incest within the realm of sexual violence. Yet, important as this is, there has been little account of how feminist work itself relates to other ways of talking about and understanding incest.

In *Interrogating Incest* Vikki Bell focuses on incest and its place in sociological theory, feminist theory and criminal law. She discusses the argument in Foucault that incest is at a point of tension between the deployment of alliance (kinship) and the deployment of sexuality. In addition, she explores how the notion of the 'incest taboo' might be worked back into the feminist understanding of incest.

By examining incest from a critical Foucauldian framework Vikki Bell considers how feminist discourse on incest itself fits into other ways of talking about sex, and offers a detailed analysis of the concepts of power and knowledge in relation to the Foucault–feminist debate. Closely surveying the historical background to incest legislation and the theoretical issues involved, she delineates the impact of the different ways of understanding incest on the shape of the legislation, and shows what uncomfortable questions and important dilemmas are raised by viewing the criminalisation of incest within the Foucauldian framework.

Vikki Bell is a Lecturer in Sociology at Goldsmiths' College, University of London.

SOCIOLOGY OF LAW AND CRIME

Editors:
Maureen Cain, *University of the West Indies*
Carol Smart, *University of Leeds*

This series presents the latest critical and international scholarship in sociology, legal theory, and criminology. Books in the series will integrate the sociology of law and the sociology of crime, extending beyond both disciplines to analyse the distribution of power. Realist, critical, and postmodern approaches will be central to the series, while the major substantive themes will be gender, class and race as they affect and, in turn, are shaped by legal relations. Throughout, the series will present fresh theoretical interpretations based on the latest empirical research. Books for early publication in the series deal with such controversial issues as child custody, criminal and penal policy, and alternative legal theory.

Titles in this series include:

CHILD CUSTODY AND THE POLITICS OF GENDER
Carol Smart and Selma Sevenhuijsen (eds)

FEMINISM AND THE POWER OF LAW
Carol Smart

OFFENDING WOMEN
Female Lawbreakers and the Criminal Justice System
Anne Worrall

FEMININITY IN DISSENT
Alison Young

JURISPRUDENCE AS IDEOLOGY
Valerie Kerruish

THE MYTHOLOGY OF MODERN LAW
Peter Fitzpatrick

First published 1993
by Routledge,
11 New Fetter Lane, London EC4P 4EE

Simultaneously published in the USA and Canada
by Routledge
29 West 35th Street, New York, NY 10001

© 1993 Vikki Bell

Typeset in Baskerville by
NWL Editorial Services, Langport, Somerset

Printed and bound in Great Britain by
T.J. Press (Padstow) Ltd, Padstow, Cornwall

British Library Cataloguing in Publication Data
A catalogue record for this book is available from the British Library.

Library of Congress Cataloging in Publication Data
Bell, Vikki, 1967 –
Interrogating incest : feminism, Foucault and the law/Vikki Bell.
p.   cm. – (Sociology of law and crime)
Includes bibliographical references and index.
1. Incest.   2. Feminist theory.   3. Sex crimes.   4. Foucault,
Michel.   I. Title.   II. Series.
HQ71.B32   1993
306.877–dc20

ISBN 0–415–07951–9
0–415–10104–2 (pbk) ✓

INTERROGATING INCEST

INCEST

Feminism, Foucault and the Law

Vikki Bell

London and New York

CONTENTS

PREFACE

> The more I read, and the more that women talked to me about their experiences, the more it became clear that not only was I looking at father–daughter rape, but also at a phenomenon of epic proportions . . . an enormous proportion of girl-children raped, molested, abused and used by their father, stepfather, de facto father, grandfather, uncle, brother; the whole hidden from view by the resounding silence of the 'incest taboo'.
>
> (Ward, 1984: 3)

This book arises out of the observation that within feminism incest has been subsumed under a discussion of sexual violence, which, whilst politically important, has meant that not much time has been spent considering how feminist work relates to other ways of talking about incest. These other 'understandings' of incest have been depicted as myths that maintain a silence about the realities of sexual abuse within the household. The notion of the incest taboo and the issue of consensual incest, which once attracted the attention of the 'founding fathers' of sociology, have been defined out of the remit of the feminist work, not because of a refusal to acknowledge their existence, but because they have not presented themselves as feminist issues. But suppose we put the feminist work 'back' into the sociological debates around incest. How would a feminist perspective refigure those sociological debates? What impact would such an exercise have on the feminist position?

In 1989 the *Sunday Mirror* reported the following case, that of a woman who

> ditched her husband and deserted her family to start a new life with her father. . . . She said: 'it seemed the most natural

thing in the world to make love'. . . . The illicit lovers survived a most terrifying trial for incest to become Britain's most bizarre couple. . . . The judge at Chelmsford Crown Court dismissed the case after [the woman's] lawyers claimed that her mother had had many other lovers who could have fathered her. . . . 'At the trial the judge warned us not to have any children. Obviously he was concerned that any child might be handicapped. I think fate made sure I had a perfect child.'

(Sunday Mirror, 5.3.1989)

What strikes me about this case is the way in which the wrong of incest is understood. The woman appeals to the powerful discourse of romantic love in her presentation of the events, stating that although 'I see now that what we did was a sin', at the time she did not see it as wrong because, from her perspective, it was not 'incest' but an instance of adult sexuality: 'It was not like father and daughter at all. He was a man and I was a woman.' The English legal system, on the other hand, is working with an understanding of incest that does not consider love or consent to be relevant issues. The dismissal of the case was not condoning their relationship but, by casting doubt on the man's paternity, denying it was incest at all. At the same time, the judge, hedging his bets, advises the couple not to have children, suggesting that, in his mind, the reason incest is wrong is because it runs a risk to any potential offspring.

For feminism, clearly, incest is wrong where it is an instance of abuse, where it is non-consensual. However, that the nature and not the quality of the relationship between the couple is the *legal* issue was brought home in a different case reported in 1990 in Scotland, where although the crime of incest is somewhat differently defined from English law, the definition similarly excludes the question of consent, defining certain relationships as incest whether the intercourse is consenting or not:

A man who served a year for incest has had his conviction quashed after genetic fingerprinting revealed that the girl was not his daughter. The man was jailed in 1986 after pleading guilty to an incestuous relationship with the girl, whom he believed to be his daughter, while she was aged 16–19. After his release from jail, the man was charged again with having unlawful sex with the girl. By that time, genetic fingerprinting techniques had become available

and tests revealed that there was no blood relationship
between them.

(The Scotsman, 8.10.1990)

By default (the tests had been conducted in order to identify
semen stains and not to establish paternity), the arrival of new
technologies in legal procedures enabled this man to challenge
his previous conviction for incest, even though no one involved
denied that intercourse had taken place and both he and the
young woman believed him to be her father.

In attempting to look at the feminist work on incestuous abuse
within the context of other ways of understanding the wrong of
incest, and with particular reference to how these understandings impinge on law, this book considers how incest is 'put
into discourse' within the 'power–knowledge–pleasure' network
that Michel Foucault made his object of study. Initially I found
Foucault's work intriguing because certain arguments seemed to
sit well with the feminist work, such as his explication of a power
that controls through the mechanism of a gaze or his insistence
that sexuality is constructed through discourse. However, in
some important senses Foucault's thesis throws down a gauntlet
to feminists hoping to break the 'conspiracy of silence' around
sexual abuse in order to emerge into a better, freer, more
understanding world. He implicitly casts the feminist work as
naive, slavishly reproducing models of understanding power and
freedom that fail to grasp the present operations of power
around sex, and thereby falling into the trap of producing more
and more talk on sex that, far from liberating us, ensnares us
deeper into the web. Thus the task became as much one of
conducting a debate between Foucault and feminism and an
investigation into the possibilities of Foucauldian feminism as it was
an investigation of the issue of incest.

In mounting such an investigation, I have had to run to keep
up with the publication of relevant texts, feeling at times, I
imagined in my more deluded moments, like Virginia Woolf in
the British Museum when faced with the enormity of her
investigation into women and fiction:

> Here had I come with a notebook and a pencil proposing to
> spend a morning reading, supposing that at the end of the
> morning I should have transferred the truth to my
> notebook. . . . 'How shall I ever find the grains of truth

embedded in all this mass of paper?' I asked myself, and in despair began running my eye up and down the long list of titles.

(1973: 28)

This book has taken four years in all to write; I have indeed read a 'mass of paper', the many sociological, feminist and legal books and articles that somehow pertain to the topic in hand. I hope the reader will therefore forgive the attempts I have made to contain the argument of this book by, for example, focusing on the first volume of Foucault's *The History of Sexuality* without discussing how the subsequent volumes changed the direction of Foucault's thought, by considering British law without discussion of other countries' legal attitudes to incest, and by locating general movements in sociology's approach to incest without detailed discussion of the contributions of specific authors. I do not claim to have disembedded the grains of truth from this area exactly, since, in Woolf's words, 'when a subject is highly controversial – and any question about sex is that – one cannot hope to tell the truth. One can only show how one came to hold whatever opinion one does hold' (1973: 6). And so I shall try. . . .

London, 1992

SERIES EDITORS' PREFACE

This text is part of a growing body of evidence that feminist scholarship in the field of law and legal theory has come of age. Feminist work in this sphere has been building on and developing from early empirical studies of the impact of law on women. These vital studies provided the grounding so essential to the work of building a scholarship which could become reflexive and self-critical. While such work remains important this book is a departure from that early tradition.

Here we find a text which has three main aims. The first is critically to document and develop feminist theories of incest. This discussion is equally valid to the student as to the teacher in that it generously evaluates competing ideas and gently moves the reader on to different ways of conceptualising the problem of incest.

The second aim is to trace the debate between Foucault and feminism. This text could be read for this alone and should become a major contribution to this continuing debate. Vikki Bell does not engage with a strawman version of Foucault but brings a depth of understanding to his work and acknowledges the shifts in his later position on power and agency. Nonetheless this is a critical evaluation, but one which suggests that feminism would be unwise to disregard Foucault's insights even where, on the face of it, they may seem antipathetical to the feminist project(s).

The third aim is to deconstruct the law of incest. Vikki Bell asks what the subject of the incest prohibition was and is. She traces the shifting arguments from their focus on 'unnatural acts', to fears of inbreeding, to concerns over harm. She is equally critical of aspects of all of these constructions. In so doing she combines feminism with Foucault to provide a new way of reading incest. This entails treating feminism as a discourse amongst other discourses and yet retaining a commitment to feminism. In this respect this text finds itself at the heart of wider debates which are occupying the attention of all 'committed' academics and political activists. The question posed is 'how can we be conscious and critical of the way in which our position is constructed whilst being critical of other accounts which we regard as less valid?'

The issue of incest, like rape, seems to give rise to 'obvious feminist truths' because of the horror these acts provoke. Here we are required to retain our commitment but to become more sceptical of such obvious truths. In this respect this contribution to the Series transcends its specific subject matter and becomes central to debates beyond law and crime. It should therefore find a wide readership from the sociology of law and criminology to women's studies and feminist theory and epistemology. This is what we mean when we say that this text is an example of a 'coming of age'.

Carol Smart and Maureen Cain
February 1993

ACKNOWLEDGEMENTS

I am pleased to have the opportunity to thank those who have helped me in the production of this book. My greatest intellectual debt is to Beverley Brown and Lynn Jamieson at Edinburgh University, whose commitment and wisdom guided me through the thesis on which this book is based. Carol Smart has maintained my momentum and enthusiasm through the last eighteen months of preparing the manuscript. Thanks also to the friends, colleagues and students who have commented on draft chapters for me. Further back, I have been encouraged and inspired by several teachers to whom I will always be grateful: my first sociology teacher, Marion Howlett, and my tutors at Cambridge, who included Kum-Kum Bhavnani, Brendan Burchell, Jenny Kitzinger and Sally Cline.

I acknowledge with love the consistent and unobstrusive support of my family, in particular my parents, Claire and David. Nathaniel and Vivian have been patient with their bookish aunt this past year. Many invaluable friends have provided encouragement as well as breaks from writing. Thanks to you all in London, Cambridge, Edinburgh, Florence and elsewhere; especially to Samantha King, Charlotte Pomery and, last but not least, Tim Kirkpatrick.

The Economic and Social Research Council funded my postgraduate studies at Edinburgh University.

1

INTRODUCTION
Interrogating incest

This book is focused on the issue of incest and its place in sociological theorising, in feminist theorising, and in British criminal law. A sociological riddle, a feminist issue and a category of law – incest is all these things. But is 'incest' the same at each of these sites? What is incest 'about' in each of the discourses in which it resides? In this chapter I will briefly sketch the problematics which provide both the inspiration for this book and the context in which it should be read: first, the feminist analyses of incestuous abuse, which have radically challenged previous sociological emphasis on the incest prohibition; secondly, the provocative work of Michel Foucault, in particular his arguments about the ways in which sex has been 'put into discourse'; and thirdly, the developments in the sociology of law and crime to which both Foucault and feminism have contributed.

INCEST, SOCIOLOGY AND FEMINISM

Incest is a topic of longstanding interest to social scientists. Over the course of a century or so, sociologists and social anthropologists have explored the incest prohibition as the example *par excellence* of a social rule. Many influential social scientists contributed to the debates around the prohibition of incest.[1] Initially, the questions posed reflected the dominant sociological interest in finding social facts and order in life. The incest prohibition was declared a safe fact, an universal social rule, and the debates took this as their point of departure, asking either 'how did the incest prohibition originate?' or 'why did societies institute such a taboo, i.e. what function does it serve?' In these discussions, the actual occurrence of incest was considered rare; where acknowledged, it was considered outside the remit of sociology, inhabiting instead the realms of abnormal psychology, where it did not contradict the sorts of questions under investigation. If sociology's task was to uncover the broad social patterns of life, it was not those who committed incest who were the focus of attention, but the majority who did not. Those who commit incest do not threaten the notion of the incest prohibition as a fundamental social rule because they are regarded not as *social* beings, but as 'misfits'. More recently, interest in the incest prohibition has begun to question the term itself, asking whether what had previously been recognised as the incest prohibition in many different societies really means the same thing in each society. Thus it has been suggested that transposing the template of 'the incest prohibition' onto all societies has conflated differences in what and who is actually forbidden (see, e.g., Goody, 1971; Ember, 1983). There is still debate on the question of the incest taboo, but this interest is one that seems to have become confined within the discipline of social anthropology. Sociology's interest in the issue of incest has turned elsewhere.

The recent 'discovery' of incest as a social problem has meant that the questions it raises for sociology have changed. Sexual abuse within the household has become acknowledged as a cause for public concern. The early 'speakouts' by women survivors revealed what had been considered a rare crime to be a widespread form of sexual abuse (Armstrong, 1978; Ward, 1984). The ensuing discussions of incest have taken place on a much more public stage than had the earlier musings of social theoreticians. Over the past decade or so, many media discussions have highlighted the issue, and in the academic arena social science no longer proffers theories of the incest prohibition. Where incest is discussed it tends to be as a social problem, sometimes alongside surveys or speculations on the extent of this problem. Thus incest seems to have changed or be in the process of changing discourse within social science. It no longer finds its place as a social rule requiring explanation as to its origin and function, but has been identified as an abusive practice, located as a social problem to be uncovered and measured.

But in the move from the emphasis on the prohibition to the emphasis on the practice, theory does not somehow get 'left behind'. Statistics and surveys need to be explained and discussed. This inevitably means placing some form of theoretical

2

framework around them. In terms of 'explaining' the occurrence of incest it has been feminist analyses, in the main, which have taken up the challenge of framing the *sociological* questions. In sociology, it would be fair to say, incest has become the preserve of feminism. It has been feminist analyses which have provided the alternative voice to individualistic explanations. Looking at the social patterning of incestuous abuse, feminists have pointed to the normality of the offenders, their families and their lives. The offenders do not fit the stereotypical image of the sexual pervert which the emphasis on the prohibition as universal and universally obeyed seemed to imply. Nor do they come from any particular class or racial background (see, e.g., La Fontaine, 1990). Feminists argue that incest is a form of sexual abuse, one that is perpetrated mainly by men, and one that has to be understood within the context of a society in which men are able to exercise power over women and children in a sexualised way. The feminist analyses place incest within the range of male violences, understanding incest on the model of the feminist understanding of rape. The various renamings of incest convey this relocation: 'incestuous assault' (Butler, 1985); 'Father– Daughter rape' (Ward, 1984).

Thus feminist work has not only challenged the sociological faith in the incest prohibition by contributing to the 'airing' of the issue and showing the extent of the problem in terms of numbers. More than this, it presents, if in the margins of feminist texts and discussions, a profound *theoretical* shift in the way in which incest is conceived in the sociological imagination. As opposed to placing incest on the side of the 'abnormal', feminist contributions suggest that, on the contrary, given the power dynamics of male-dominated society and the understandings of sexuality which we live out, incestuous abuse is in a sense unsurprising. In feminist analysis, incest signals not the chaos it did (and does) for sociological functionalism, but an order, the familiar and familial order of patriarchy, in both its strict and its feminist sense. Incest reveals the gendered power dynamics of the society in which we exist. Importantly, feminists argue that incest cannot be regarded as *asocial* at all, but has to be analysed instead in direct relation to the social structures which are continually produced and reproduced as 'normal'. Turning the earlier sociological discussions on their head, therefore, feminists argue that it is not the incest prohibition but, rather, the actual occurrence of incest which provides a key to a sociological understanding of social structure and culture.[2]

SHIFTING THEORETICAL GROUND: RADICAL
FEMINISM AND MICHEL FOUCAULT

This book is an attempt to look at a number of theoretical questions which cluster around the issue of incest. Whilst sympathetic to the feminist discourse that situates incest as a form of sexual violence, I want to consider incest from within a different theoretical framework from the one in which it is usually placed by feminism. Previous feminist analyses of incest have tended to be directed at exposing the occurrence of incest as a form of sexual abuse perpetrated by men. This is their immediate aim. But as I have suggested, these works are by no means 'untheoretical'. They use and create concepts that are theoretical, and present arguments within a framework of understanding that cannot be other than theoretical. This theoretical framework tends to be a radical feminist one. I label it so because these works have all the hallmarks of radical feminism. The arguments are firmly rooted in women's experiences, exposing the collective experiences of many women, and, through presenting the similarities in those experiences, drawing the conclusion that incest is a *political* matter. It is an example of the personal is political in the sense that although incestuous abuse has been and is experienced by women as a personal matter, a matter of which they can speak to no one, it is in fact about relations of power between groups: between men and women, and between men and children, particularly in the context of the institution of the family.

One of the tasks of this book is to investigate the theoretical stance taken by feminists writing on incest. I do so by considering its relation to debates which have been taking place within feminist theory and feminist analyses of law. In particular, I consider how the feminist analyses of incest relate to the recent feminist interest in the usefulness of the work of French philosopher Michel Foucault.

Foucault was by no means a feminist writer. A concern with women's oppression barely flickers in the vast majority of his writings. So what is it about Foucault's work that makes it worthy of such extended excavation within a feminist study? An easy answer would be simply that Foucault's work has become widely read and used in malestream sociological work. The fact that Foucault's work has covered many different subjects – medicine,

4

madness, prisons, sexuality – has meant that it has been incorporated into several disciplines. He has been regarded as an innovative and exciting writer, if frustrating in his obscurity and his refusal to situate his work within the literature of the disciplines in which he is writing. Thus Foucault has become integrated into the social science of which feminist social theory forms a part. In that sense feminist exploration of his arguments is of 'obvious' interest and importance.

There are, however, more specific reasons why Foucault's arguments are of interest for feminist analyses. These relate to the content of Foucault's work, to the subject areas with which his work, and particularly his later work, was concerned. Here one finds the terms which highlight common ground between Foucault and feminism: sexuality, power and knowledge. Of these three principal themes, it is the first two which most clearly coincide with feminist concerns. *Sexuality* has been a focus of much feminist writing, and, in particular, of radical feminist work. There is now a growing body of feminist work which discusses the ways in which women's sexuality is policed, denied, exploited, as a means of the social control of women. Sexuality has been posited as a, if not the, central site of women's oppression. In the context of sexual abuse, feminist analyses have increasingly focused on the social construction of male (hetero)sexuality as a crucial component of feminist theorising. *Power* is also a central concept in feminist analyses. Exposing, exploring and changing the ways in which men, both individually and as a group, exercise power over women might pass relatively uncontroversially as a definition of the feminist task. The third term that I have assigned to Foucault's work, that of *knowledge*, may be less clearly a feminist term. Yet the study of knowledge is certainly a concern of feminism, one of increasing debate in theoretical areas, but also in the more classical radical feminist mode of challenging 'myths' that prevail in our society, e.g. myths around women's nature, motherhood, sexuality, or, indeed, myths around incest.

Having indicated a concurrence of subject areas on some general level, one must immediately note that there are also particular theoretical problems in bringing Foucault's work into feminist discussions. Some feminist writers have found Foucault's work highly problematic for feminist inquiry. His work on power has been described as 'inadequate and even irrelevant' to the needs of feminism (Hartsock, 1990: 166). His work on discourse has been said to 'deprive [women] of the conceptual weapons with which they can understand and begin to overcome their subordination' (Balbus, 1982: 476). Danger warnings to those feminists who use Foucault are not infrequent. Are these warnings to pass unheeded? My stance is as follows. Whilst there are certainly some points of conflict that require discussion, lest a feminist utilisation of Foucault become unprincipled eclecticism, I believe the following chapters illustrate not the complete convergence of opinion, for that is not my goal, but how the work of Foucault can be useful in developing a feminist understanding of social processes in a way that does not take on his ideas at the expense of leaving feminist insights behind.

This study is not the first to suggest a use of Foucault in this sympathetic but critical way. His work has already been explored by several feminist writers. There have been articles, books and edited collections which use Foucault in a feminist context. But incest has not previously been a subject on which Foucault and feminism have been brought together. Indeed, the issue of incest does not seem the most obvious terrain on which to explore the work of Foucault and its relation to feminist thought. Partly this is so because radical feminism tends to be regarded as the most separatist strand of feminism, including separate from male dominance in academic texts. It is the strand which has most loudly declared that feminist work should stem from women's experiences, remain 'accessible' and hence not get entangled with theory. Since incestuous abuse and sexual violence in general have been addressed mainly by radical feminist writers, incest might seem an unlikely subject on which to link feminism with the work of Foucault. It is also partly because what Foucault did say about child sexual abuse feminists would find objectionable. In *The History of Sexuality Volume 1: An Introduction* he refers to what feminists would regard as an instance of child sexual abuse as 'these inconsequential bucolic pleasures' (1981: 33).

Nevertheless, the feminist analyses of incest have the ingredients that I have suggested form common ground between feminist theorists and Foucault, being concerned with sexuality, power and knowledge. Illustrating how the arguments of the feminist writers on incest frequently can be seen to dovetail with arguments that are taking place in other, more obviously theoretical and seemingly contrasting, feminist arenas is one of the most challenging and exciting aspects of this study.

DEVIANCE, FOUCAULT AND FEMINIST ANALYSES OF LAW

I have drawn a sketch of a movement from early macro-sociological concern with social cohesion and the incest prohibition as a social fact to concerns with social problems and consideration of the social patterning of incestuous practice, the latter being prompted primarily by feminist concern and discussed in that context. Echoes of this pattern can be found in the trajectory that has been sketched by Cohen and Scull (1985) in relation to the sociology of deviance and crime. According to Cohen and Scull, the sociological task began with issues of social control in a wide sense. Thus Durkheim, for example, was interested in 'the great problem of "social order"' (Cohen and Scull, 1985: 5). His work was concerned with the way in which society functions in a relatively orderly fashion without the need for explicitly coercive intervention. He argued that society continually reflects its social morals and norms back to itself, and that this was crucial in producing the self-regulating order that was his object of analysis.

What happened in the twentieth century, according to Cohen and Scull, was a move away from these large-scale questions about the order of society toward an emphasis on how the individual joins this order. This gave sociological questions a distinct social psychological slant. The issues were different from the issue of social control in Durkheim's sense, or, for that matter, the similarly macro-scale problematics in Marx's or Weber's work. The concept of social control was reinterpreted such that it moved away from its original connotations of 'order, authority, power and social organisation' and became the question of how individuals come to fit into this ordered society; thus 'the emphasis was on the *processes* of the individual's induction into society – that is, the problem of socialisation' (Cohen and Scull, 1985: 5, original emphasis).

Thus, in the sociology of crime and deviance, there was a shift 'downwards', away from the ambitious Durkheimian questions of social facts and group processes to questions of the social processes that produce the individual 'deviant'. Studies which traced the problem of delinquency 'backwards' to 'poor parenting', 'broken' homes or educational underachievement are examples of this focus on socialisation as the central issue in sociology. These explanations of crime and deviance had the effect of isolating sociological questions about crime from sociological questions about the role of the state making 'the family' or 'the peer group' the focus of attention (Cohen and Scull, 1985: 6).

Cohen and Scull suggest that from the late 1960s onwards work in the area of the sociology of crime and deviance has returned to more macro-sociological questions. In the socio-historical context of the radical politics of the era, criminologists and sociologists began to consider the question 'who decides and enforces what is criminal?' Although never accepted as a complete theoretical explanation of crime, Becker's (1963) labelling theory presented the possibility that the definitions of crime and the processes by which these definitions are policed and enforced is crucial. This (re)turned the attention of sociologists 'upwards' towards concepts of authority, power and the state, the macro-questions of early sociology. Joining with the scepticism of radical movements in psychiatry, social work and medicine, the sociology of deviance has since incorporated the study of how crime and deviance are defined, thereby incorporating historical, economic and political processes into its field of vision. Socio-legal issues, the study of how the law operates as a *social* institution, have become reunited with questions of the commission of 'deviant acts'.

One author who has been highly influential in this (re)turning to questions of definition, power and the state is Michel Foucault. His *Discipline and Punish* (1979a) has been widely read and drawn upon in this area since it concerns questions of power in the history of the prison (amongst other institutions) and questions of how deviants and criminals are defined and written about. Foucault discusses the relationship between the operations of power and the production of knowledge in a way which implicates the sociology of deviance and crime just as much as more policy-oriented knowledges. In *The History of Sexuality Volume 1: An Introduction* (1981) Foucault continues this mode of inquiry, this time looking at the ways in which power both operates to produce knowledges of sexual practices and operates within those knowledges. Foucault's work is ambitious in its historical scope and provocative in its forthright arguments. Along with other, very different writers, his work has thus been part of the relatively recent shift 'up' (to questions of definitions) but also 'out' (to questions of politics and economics) and 'back' (to historical questions).

In their review of the sociology of crime and deviance, Cohen and Scull fail to mention feminism as an important influence. Feminists have been writing in the field of crime and deviance since the mid-1970s, critiquing the 'gender-blindness' of the mainstream theories that have been put forward. But further-more, feminists have highlighted, as they have in the social sciences more generally, the importance of taking a wider political perspective, of looking at definitions of what behaviour is and what behaviour is not acceptable. The response to sexual abuse is a case in point. The ways in which the sexual abuse of girls and women is shrugged off as 'having a bit of fun', the result of her 'tempting' the man, etc., have been well documented in the feminist literature (e.g. Wilson, 1983; Stanko, 1985). Feminists have argued that the response to sexual abuse by the police and criminal justice system reflects and reproduces that which sexual abuse receives outside law: sexual abuse has been treated not as a criminal offence, but, in the words of one judge earlier this century, as 'the sort of thing that might happen to any man' (Jeffreys, 1985: 55).[3] Whilst recent changes have improved police and legal procedures, there is still a healthy scepticism arising out of the fear that these may prove cosmetic on some levels. Arguably, therefore, feminism has played a significant part in the developments in the sociology of deviance and crime that Cohen and Scull describe and must be credited as part of the force behind the current sociological interest in issues of social control, in questions about how crime is defined and policed.

Of course, these influences on the sociology of crime do not take place in isolation from one another. Thus, as one would expect, there has also been some 'sideways' influence between Foucault and feminism. Whilst feminism's influence on Foucault's work was probably slight – as I have already mentioned, he never seemed to respond to feminism and never did he espouse feminist ideals – there has been, as well as the general interest discussed above, feminist interest in Foucault in the area of the sociology of law, crime and deviance. In particular, the work of Carol Smart (1989) has argued that Foucault's work can be of use in furthering the feminist theorising of law, precisely because it pro-vides discussion of the operations of power, knowledge and processes of definition that can be seen at work in and around law.

Smart argues that feminist analyses should work to de-centre law; many feminist perspectives have conceded too much to law, accepting its importance in the feminist struggle without questioning why it should be so central. But law is only central and important to the extent that we accept its self-definition. It is this self-definition that Smart suggests feminists need to interrogate. The perspective which Smart adopts is a Foucauldian one. She regards the law as a discourse which has a privileged position from which to exercise power. Within the parameters of the legal method, the law 'is able to refute and disregard alternative discourses and to claim a special place in the definition of events' (1989: 162). The argument is that although other knowledges and other interpretations of events are articulated both within the legal process and outside law, they are only selectively 'heard'. The law exercises its power to disqualify knowledges and definitions of events through the notion of a legal method. Frequently, other knowledge is heard only to the extent that it can be recast as pertinent to *legal* issues. If not, it is excluded. For example, in a rape case, the woman's knowledge of events is only 'heard' when it touches upon what the law sees as relevant. (One might also add that the legal method can highlight aspects of the situation that the woman does not see as important in the train of events, e.g. that she knew this man before, that she had had consensual intercourse with him before, etc.) The Truth that is propounded in any particular case, therefore, is based upon a method which establishes the law's status as knowledge and the legal personnel as experts.

The law is often confronted with other discourses in society such as medical, social work, or even feminist discourse. Smart suggests that the law invites these other discourses onto its territory, thus creating tensions around which is to define the Truth of events. Smart suggests that there can be no easy predictions of what happens in such a situation; sometimes the law defers to another discourse, allowing it to have significant entry to legal decisions, but at others, the law colonises the other discourse, and reinterprets the knowledges propounded there in terms of legal language. In the latter case, the law extends its traditional power by incorporating arenas initially the terrain of others into the legal domain. This is particularly the case with the discourses of the 'psy' professionals (psychologists, social workers, etc.). The example Smart discusses here is that of reproductive technologies. Whilst medicine has created the possibility of different types of relationships by breaking the traditional associations between the production of eggs, giving birth and social motherhood as well as traditional associations between women and men in this context, the law has been concerned with drawing up the surrounding legal issues such as the ownership of frozen embryos. In doing so, it establishes itself as a knowledge which can be drawn upon when such cases arrive in court. Smart's thesis is that the power of law lies in its ability to set itself up as holding the key to Truth. How law comes to be regarded as having access to the Truth, the processes by which law allows or disallows interpretations of events, and how law extends its terrain into traditionally non-legal discourses – these are the questions which need to occupy feminist perspectives on law.

In this book I want to shadow the general move that has been made in the area of sociology of crime, to explore recent feminist work on incest as a theoretical and political contribution to the sociology of crime, and to feed this work back into wider sociological questions of power, knowledge and the law. To some extent the feminist work on incest already points in this direction, arguing as it does that the commission of incest is not an individual problem of individual men, the result of poor or problematic socialisation, but is about wider questions of power and of sexuality in our society. But there has been little discussion of how feminist discussions of incest as a social problem relate to how the incest prohibition has been theorised, nor to criminal law on incest, where we find the most stark prohibition in the classic form of 'thou shalt not'. This is the move this book attempts.

In a sense, the 'route' by which I make this move is via the work of Michel Foucault. His work is a pivot around which to situate my discussions for the reasons I have discussed. His work clusters around terms that are of great importance to feminist analyses (power, sexuality, knowledge), including, if not especially, radical feminist work such as that which has addressed the issue of incestuous abuse; he figures importantly in the general broadening away from micro-sociological concerns in the area of deviance (back) towards macro sociological questions of power, law and the state; moreover, he has been influential in feminist analyses of law, in particular the recent work of Carol Smart (1989).

OUTLINE OF THE BOOK

There are therefore a number of intersecting debates which this book brings together. These are debates which concern different areas of social science. As a consequence, the chapters focus on different questions around incest. It is my intention that each of the chapters be sufficiently independent to enable the reader to dip into the one which touches upon her or his interests, but that the more general arguments are ones which will be built through the book as a whole.

In Chapter 2 I take space to discuss the broad theoretical relationship between feminist theorising and the work of Foucault, in particular his *The History of Sexuality Volume 1: An Introduction*. Rather than rehearse the commonalities between Foucault and feminism, I focus instead upon the problems of bringing them together. By working through what appear to be the 'stumbling blocks' between Foucault and feminism, I seek to build a considered theoretical stance on the possibilities of a feminist/Foucauldian approach. Chapter 3 comes back to the specific issue of incest, taking a detailed look at the arguments that feminists have made around the issue of incest, and suggesting how a Foucauldian perspective might operate in the clarification of these feminist arguments. My purpose here is not to suggest that the feminist work is 'wrong', but to suggest where Foucault's ideas become relevant to this feminist work. Exploring the interconnections it appears that feminist work is often already asking similar questions to Foucault such that bringing the two together operates to draw out the theoretical implications of the feminist perspective. Thus I intend not to collapse the feminist position into a Foucauldian perspective but to elevate its particular contributions through the challenges presented by Foucault's work.

In a sense Chapter 4 makes a similar manoeuvre, but this time it begins from within the Foucauldian framework in an investigation of Foucault's comments on the topic of incest. Foucault situates incest at a pivotal point in the thesis of *The History of Sexuality*, placing it between the 'old' and the 'new' ways of talking about sex. I consider how feminist discourse fits into these ways of talking about incest, and how the 'old' ways of talking about incest, predominantly talk about the incest prohibition, relates to feminist work. I argue that the incest prohibition holds an ambiguous place in feminist work, sometimes rejected outright, sometimes reworked. Drawing on Foucault's arguments and those of Judith Butler (1990a), I extend the feminist critique of the notion of an incest prohibition, suggesting that the incest taboo exists 'only' as a discursive rule.

One place in which the incest prohibition is clearly 'put into discourse' is in criminal law. In the stark form of 'thou shalt not' incest is criminalised in both English and Scots law. In Chapter 5, I investigate this criminalisation through consideration of the parliamentary debates that shaped the crime of incest as it presently appears on the statute books. I argue that the legal pronouncement relies upon several different ways of under-standing incest, including the newer bio-political knowledges surrounding sex. Using a Foucauldian approach and framework, therefore, I extend the feminist/Foucauldian argument offered in Chapter 4, i.e. that the incest prohibition is a discursive phenomenon. This is not just to say that it exists insofar as we talk about it, but that it is upheld through a cluster of discursive practices, with different points of articulation, that converge to create and sustain the prohibition. I suggest that the criminalisation of incest has to be understood as an example of recreating the incest prohibition, an 'old' way of talking about incest, through the voicing of predominantly 'new' ways of talking about incest, i.e. the bio-political knowledges. This argument extends the feminist perspective on law offered by Smart (1989). Chapter 6 considers and critiques the arguments made by Foucault in two separate debates. The first is a debate about the de-criminalisation of sexual relationships between adults and children. I argue that whilst Foucault appears to think his policy position follows from his theoretical position, the move he makes is not necessarily the only logical conclusion implied by his work. I argue that the radical theoretical position would not translate into a radical position in practice; in fact, it would in all probability be a conservative move. The crux of this discussion is the important question of consent. The second is a debate about rape in which Foucault suggests that it be treated as a violent crime and not as a sexual one. Finally, Chapter 7 reflects upon the issues raised in the book, reviewing the implications of the theoretical manoeuvres and the questions that remain problematic.

2

A CONTINUAL CONTEST
Foucault and feminism

[R]ather than a marriage or a new political school, we would
say that the convergences of feminism and Foucault suggest
the possibility of a friendship grounded in political and
ethical commitment.

(Diamond and Quinby, 1988: ix)

To the question whether a Foucauldian feminism is a
contradiction in terms, a Foucauldian feminist might reply;
'No, not a contradiction but a continual contestation.'

(Sawicki, 1988: 176)

Feminist theory has often been in the position of responding to
male social theorists, be it within the context of Marxism,
liberalism or psychoanalysis. In exploring the work of Michel
Foucault, perhaps this book will be pigeon-holed as yet another
instance of this recurrent pattern, as still caught within the
heterosexual matrix of a feminist responding to the work of a
'great' male thinker. Of course it will be for the reader to judge
whether this is ultimately what this work does. For my part, I do
not consider the argument to be concerned with why feminism
needs Foucault. His work is not the source of all answers to
feminist questions and it is not the intention to set up Foucault as
an infallible authority; my aim is instead to extract those parts of
his work which are pertinent to feminist inquiry in search of a
productive dialogue.

Feminist theory is a diverse and contradictory body of knowledge such that instigating a conversation between 'feminism' and
Foucault is bound to draw selectively on the literature available.
Moreover, since there is now a substantial body of feminist work
which draws upon Foucault, the journey has already been

14

charted somewhat. It is, nevertheless, a worthwhile exercise to lay out the parameters of both the 'possible friendship' and the 'continual contestation' between Foucault and feminism. In this chapter, therefore, I want to put the specific focus on incest to one side and take space to explore these broad theoretical issues. There are three terms or themes around which feminism and Foucault converge and which are of import to the issues raised in this book as a whole: sexuality, power and knowledge. Because these themes are addressed most directly by Foucault in *The History of Sexuality Volume 1: An Introduction* (1981) the chapter will concentrate primarily upon this work (hereafter *THS*). I approach the question of how Foucault's work may be of interest to feminism through a consideration of these themes, and through discussion of the potential stumbling blocks to a Foucauldian feminism.

SEXUALITY

In *THS*, Foucault takes it as read that sexuality is socially constructed. At its most general, the 'social constructionist' perspective holds that sexuality is not a property of the body, nor a natural tendency, but is formed within and informed by the society in which one lives. This type of analysis is not unfamiliar in sociological work, and is one that much feminist work on sexuality adheres to (e.g. Jackson, 1978; Vance, 1984; Barale, 1986). However, to suggest that both Foucault and feminism adopt a 'social constructionist' perspective does not actually tell us much about their contributions nor about their relationship, for there is a broad range of sociological, historical and anthropological theories that belong in the melting pot of 'social constructionist' perspectives, and, as Carole Vance has suggested, the common denominator of this work is a very broad one:

> all reject transhistorical and transcultural definitions of sexuality and suggest instead that sexuality is mediated by historical and cultural factors.
>
> (1992: 134)

Thus it is important to draw out Foucault's specific contribution before one can discuss its relevance, disruptions and shortfalls with respect to feminist work. Foucault's project was to trace the history of the social construction of sexuality, to consider how sexuality has been variously and differentially produced through a study of the discourses which, he contends, surround and create sexuality. In short, *THS* is about the operations of power and the formation of knowledges about sex.

THS begins by refuting the history of sexuality as it has been habitually told, a history that depicts a move from a time in which sex was freely seen and spoken about, to a time of repression, associated with nineteenth-century prudery, when sex reputedly became a matter of shame, to be 'hidden away' in the conjugal bedroom, to, finally, the present era in which sexuality is beginning again to be liberated. It is only now, this story suggests, in the latter half of the twentieth century, that sexual liberation is beginning again to be possible.[1] To this account, Foucault contrasts his own. He argues that sexuality did not undergo a period of repression in the last century; sexuality was not silenced, but, rather, it was a time that witnessed an explosion of discourses around sex.

The thesis of *THS* is not to deny totally the repressive hypothesis that views the history of sexuality as following the trajectory 'freedom–repression–limited freedom' but to place it within a wider framework, that is, 'the emergence of multiple discourses on sexuality and the particular style of those discourses' (Cousins and Hussain, 1984: 204). The explosion of discourses to which Foucault points are not simply those of scandalous literature, those that are regularly held up as the other side of a Victorian hypocrisy around sex, but also the medical/ psychological/welfare discourses that emerged in force at this time, the knowledges that Foucault sees as forming the 'will to know'[2] about sex. In these discourses sex became something that had to be managed. It called for analytic discourses, useful and public discourses (1981: 24–5).

Any 'repression' of sexuality did not silence discourses of sex, since sex was still everywhere present even where it was expressly forbidden, in the architectural layout of schools, for example, where children were segregated according to sex by the design, entering the buildings through different doors and climbing separate staircases. Any restrictions on the way people could speak about sex was, Foucault suggests, 'only the counter-part of other discourses, and perhaps necessary in order for them to function' (1981: 30). Thus the restrictions on speaking about sex effectively created the space for knowledges of sex to be expounded by those who could 'really know' the secrets and dangers of sex (1981: 30).

> It is true that a long standing 'freedom' of language between children and adults, pupils or teachers, may have disappeared. . . . But this was not a plain and simple imposition of silence. Rather, it was a new regime of discourses. Not any less was said . . . on the contrary. But things were said in a different way; it was different people who said them, from different points of view, and in order to obtain different results. Silence itself . . . is less the absolute limit of discourse, the other side from which it is separated by a strict boundary, than an element that functions alongside the things said, with them and in relation to them within over-all strategies.
>
> (1981: 27)

Foucault's argument is developed, as Cousins and Hussain (1984: 208) note, along two lines. First, it considers the style of discourses on sexuality, and secondly, it considers the objects of these discourses. In relation to the style of discourse, Foucault argues, sexuality has been brought into the realm of knowledge, the play of true and false. It has been made a scientific concern – 'scientia sexualis' – whereby 'an entire machinery for producing true discourses concerning [sex]' is put into operation. The deployment of sexuality 'consists in strategies of relations of forces supporting, and supported by, types of knowledge' (Foucault, in Merquoir, 1985: 123). Sex is regarded as harbouring a fundamental secret that must be brought out into the open and deciphered for what it can tell of the person by those with the appropriate expertise.

Foucault's argument is that although sexuality is apparently the object of these discourses, it is itself developed through them. Foucault's interest is in the way discursive strategies 'implanted' sexuality by talking and acting in the name of a knowledge of sex. That is, it was not the target but the product of their operations:

> '[S]exuality': the correlative of that slowly developed discursive practice which constitutes the scientia sexualis. The essential features of this sexuality are not the

17

expression of a representation that is more or less distorted by ideology, or of a misunderstanding caused by taboos; they correspond to the functional requirements of a discourse that must produce its truth . . . sexuality was defined as being 'by nature': a domain susceptible to pathological processes, and hence calling for therapeutic or normalising intervention; a field of meanings to decipher; the site of processes concealed by specific mechanisms; a focus of indefinite causal relations; and an obscure speech (parole) that had to be ferreted out and listened to.

(1981: 68)

Foucault suggests that there were four great strategies relating to sexuality. He identifies these as follows: the hysterisation of women's bodies; a pedagogisation of children's sex; a social-isation of procreative behaviour; and a psychiatrisation of perverse pleasure. Emerging through these strategies were the four objects of knowledge and anchorage points for that knowledge: the hysterical woman; the masturbating child; the Malthusian couple; and the perverse adult (1981: 104). Foucault argues that through these strategies sexuality was deployed. For example, children became the focus of attention as masturbation was simultaneously spoken of as a natural inclination and as a danger, both physical and moral, individual and collective. It was asserted that 'practically all children indulge or are prone to indulge in sexual activity; and that, being unwarranted, at the same time "natural" and "contrary to nature", this sexual activity posed physical and moral, individual and collective dangers' (1981: 104). Around the child gathered 'parents, families, educators, doctors and eventually psychologists' (1981: 104) who watched out for any signs of sexuality. For the 'perverse adult', sexual acts that were previously considered simply as acts 'against nature' were now linked with something deeper, regarded as the signs of a sexuality that was pathological and in need of correction. Knowledges of homosexuality and of various other sexual 'perversions' sought to discover the cause of the abnor-mality and thereby to understand these sexual deviants.

By focusing on the 'periphery', Foucault argues, a knowledge of the normal was also built up. This argument echoes that advanced in *Discipline and Punish* (1979a), where he considered the normalising effects of penal techniques of control that simultaneously formed a knowledge of the delinquent as a type and a knowledge of the 'normal' from whose standards the inmates deviated. The strategies of the deployment of sexuality operate in a productive and normalising fashion in the sense that out of their operations an understanding of what sexuality is and what sexuality should be was formed. Foucault argues:

> What was at issue in these strategies? A struggle against sexuality? Or were they part of an effort to gain control of it? An attempt to regulate it more effectively and mask its more indiscreet, conspicuous, and intractable aspects? A way of formulating only that measure of knowledge that was acceptable and useful? In actual fact, what was involved, rather, was the very production of sexuality. Sexuality must not be thought of as a kind of natural given which power tries to hold in check, or as an obscure domain which knowledge tries gradually to uncover. It is the name that can be given to a historical construct; not a furtive reality that is difficult to grasp, but a great surface network in which the stimulation of bodies, the intensification of pleasures, the incitement to discourse, the formation of special knowledges, the strengthening of controls and resistances, are linked to one another, in accordance with a few major strategies of knowledge and power.
>
> (1981: 105–6)

Thus where traditional histories might have seen a repression of sex, or, in a Reichian-Marxist history, the elimination of non-productive sex ('work, don't make love', as Foucault remarks: 1988: 112), Foucault argues there was an incitement to talk about sex, and the very production of something we now call and generally understand as natural: sexuality. The efforts that might have been taken as signs of repression, signs of a prudery around sex, were actually, Foucault contends, about the production of that to which they were supposedly opposed. Sexuality, as we now understand the term, was being produced through a regime of 'power–knowledge–pleasure' that sustains the proliferation of discourses (1981: 11).

Not only do people in the West speak of sexuality as a natural part of ourselves, we live in a time when sexuality is regarded as a key to our inner selves. The sexual confession, long a part of Christian tradition, has taken on a new context within the twentieth century, principally around the practices of psycho-analysis. Sexuality has become part of a diffuse causality for one's problems, and the confession a clinical procedure which, with the aid of an interpreter, has positive effects for the confessor (1981: 65–7). The confession is one of the mechanisms of the deployment of sexuality, Foucault suggests, employed within many different kinds of relationships, forming a procedure by which individuals produce discourse on sexuality generally at the same time as they speak of their own particular sexual feelings, sensations and fantasies. It is Foucault's 'general working hypothesis' that

> The society that emerged in the nineteenth century – bourgeois, capitalist, or industrial society, call it what you will – did not confront sex with a fundamental refusal of recognition. On the contrary, it put into operation an entire machinery for producing true discourses concerning it. Not only did it speak of sex and compel every one to do so; it also set out to formulate the uniform truth of sex. As if it suspected sex of harbouring a fundamental secret. . . . As if it was essential that sex be inscribed not only in an economy of pleasure but in an ordered system of knowledge. . . . Thus sex gradually became an object of great suspicion.
>
> (1981: 69)

The proliferation of 'true discourses' around sexuality impinges upon our understanding of ourselves, on our subject-ivity. 'Between each of us and our sex, the West has placed a never ending demand for truth. . . . In the space of a few centuries, a certain inclination has led us to direct the question of what we are, to sex' (1981: 77–8). Foucault's work addressed questions about how we understand ourselves as sexual beings and as subjects in a more general sense. His broad argument with regard to sexuality is that we understand our sexuality through the discourses that our society makes available to us. By employing these discourses and the practices that circulate them, we embroil ourselves in the power/knowledge networks of the deployment of sexuality.

In THS there are arguments on the construction of sexuality that are specifically Foucault's as opposed to being general 'social constructionist' arguments, and which it will be useful to examine here by way of summary before exploring how they relate to feminism. Foucault's argument is that sex has become spoken about *ad nauseam* in the West; it was the eighteenth and nineteenth centuries which witnessed the beginning of this 'discursive explosion'. Foucault's interest is not so much in any talk of sex, however, but in the way in which sex has become the focus of *knowledges* which make use of 'scientific' methods in order to make truth claims about sex. Moreover, he argues, these knowledges have made a discursive move that has meant that sexual acts are regarded no longer as simply bodily acts but as acts which express 'sexuality'. Thus we now talk of someone's sexuality as though it were an essence embedded deep within her or him. Further, the knowledges have created categories of sexuality such as the 'homosexual', or 'paedophiliac', or the many categories Havelock Ellis described. Some of these categories have survived in common parlance, some only in clinical 'knowledge'; some have been adopted by those they define and 'reversed' to have positive meaning. Although these knowledges of sex have focused on the 'abnormal', they do not only have consequence for those so labelled since through the 'normalising' effect they have created a knowledge of 'normal' sexuality as well as the 'abnormal'. Scientific knowledge enters the broader discourse of sexuality such that, for example, the notion that sexual acts express an essence, 'sexuality', that is fixed and stable is presently the hegemonic 'common sense' understanding of sexuality, reproduced in everyday discourse. These knowledges are set in operation around the family as agents of 'pastoral care' watch over sexual practices. They are therefore very powerful, developed through techniques of power and deploying relations of power where they are drawn upon. Thus we can speak of the 'power/knowledge networks' of the deployment of sexuality.

So how do Foucault's arguments on sexuality relate to feminist tasks and texts? This is a difficult question because whilst feminists have been writing and working on sexuality in parallel with Foucault, the ideas presented in *THS* have also been influential in feminist circles. Nevertheless, there are clearly points of convergence and points of conflict.

Feminist work on sexuality has also considered knowledges of sexuality as pervasive and powerful tools of power. The feminist critique has attacked the supposed experts in the field of sexuality for their inaccurate or blatantly misogynist pronouncements. This critique has focused on two areas: knowledges around woman's pleasure in heterosexual relations and the way in which lesbian women have been depicted. The question 'how do women experience sexual pleasure?' has been asked over and over, leading to the production of knowledge, with 'experts' proclaiming 'the answers'. Scientific knowledge has continually positioned women's sexual pleasure as difficult and complex; 'experts' have sought to understand female sexual pleasure, principally by attempting to locate 'the site' of women's pleasure. In doing so they have until recently regarded heterosexuality as the natural and normal sexuality for women, thereby tying women to men. Sexual 'knowledge' has repeatedly described lesbians as unnatural, perverse, immature, and so on. Battles against the homophobia of 'common sense' sexual understandings are identified in lesbian and feminist texts as battles against forms of knowledge which can exert pervasive powerful effects. Thus feminists have been describing, in parallel with Foucault, the social construction of sexuality through an interrogation of powerful knowledges.

However, to suggest that feminism and Foucault are in complete harmony here is misleading, for there are also important differences in their work. In the earlier work on women's sexual pleasure, feminists tended to utilise a notion of a true and free sexuality repressed somewhere under the weight of both men's and women's ignorance of the female body. Borrowing from Foucault, Segal has criticised such work for its implication that if misogynistic and homophobic knowledges are criticised and removed it will be possible for women to find sexual pleasure and their 'true sexuality'. This is an implication she locates in several feminist texts.

> Because women's sexuality had been, as of course it had, defined in male terms, feminists have argued for some 'natural' or 'authentic' female sexuality, which we need to 'rediscover' . . . 'when we reclaim our sexuality, we will have reclaimed our belief in ourselves as women'.
>
> (Segal, 1992: 119)

Segal suggests that this is an untenable assumption, one that works with a naive perception of sexuality as natural and a liberatory force.

More recent feminist work, however, has begun to speak about how sexuality is shaped by social convention and social 'knowledge'. This perspective is clear in feminist work on male sexual violence, for example, where the social construction of masculine sexuality has taken centre stage (Edwards, 1987). Feminists note the ways in which 'normal' masculine sexuality is spoken about as aggressive, spontaneous and overpowering, and suggest that the ways in which we talk about and represent sexuality inform behaviour. Moreover, feminists suggest that the line separating 'normal' male sexuality and abusive male behaviour is a fine one. Both are informed by the same knowledges, the same 'common sense' arguments about male sexual behaviour.

The understanding of sexuality as an innate driving force emanating from within is a particularly powerful 'common sense' knowledge, and one which has had damaging consequences for women survivors of sexual violence. The feminist accounts suggest that this understanding of men's sexuality has both a *causal* effect, in that it informs men's sexuality, including the sexuality of the man who sexually abuses, and consequences *after* the abuse, informing the abuser's rationalisations of the abuse as well as others' understandings of his actions (e.g. in the 'he just couldn't help himself' argument).

On surveying the ways in which women's sexual pleasure has been described, the realities of married life, the homophobic nature of our culture and the way in which women have been positioned within discourses of male sexuality, feminist work has identified 'compulsory heterosexuality' (Rich, 1980) as an *institution*. This is a concept which differentiates feminism from the Foucauldian perspective. According to the feminist account, compulsory heterosexuality functions to persuade women by both harsh and gentle tactics into monogamous heterosexual relationships. The tactics which so persuade women have been the focus of much feminist work in this area. The marketing of 'romantic love' is a mass industry in the West, providing substance for the dreams of young girls through the one formula: 'find a man, keep him'. Work on the sexuality of young girls has shown how schoolgirls' heterosexuality is discursively policed as they negotiate the dangers of being labelled as either 'loose' or 'tight' (Lees, 1986). Lesbians have been subjected to all varieties of psychological knowledge, since they are regarded as always in need of explanation (Kitzinger, 1987). Feminist work on sexual violence has noted how the 'well founded fear' of sexual assault on the street means women enter into a relationship with a 'protective male'. This notion that men will protect women works in turn to make women reliant upon men (and to make women in domestic violence situations feel trapped, isolated and failures) (Hanmer and Saunders, 1984).

The wealth of these various contributions has enabled MacKinnon (1982) to suggest that the social formation of sexuality has to be the central process to which feminists turn their attention: it is the 'lynchpin' of gender oppression. MacKinnon suggests, furthermore, that it is through learning to be heterosexual that women learn to be 'feminine', to be recognised as 'women'.

> Socially, femaleness means femininity, which means attractiveness to men, which means sexual attractiveness, which means sexual availability on male terms.
>
> (1982: 531)

Thus the institution of heterosexuality and the ways in which it is policed and maintained has been set up as the root cause of women's problems in the realm of sexuality (and by MacKinnon as the cause of women's oppression *tout court*). In doing so, feminism locates a source or 'matrix' of oppression that seems to contrast with Foucault's emphasis on mobile and changing networks of power. Foucault's *THS* suggests that bringing everything back to an underlying cause – such as the institution of heterosexuality – may be too reductive an explanation of all operations of power around sex. Furthermore, it is perhaps due to this depiction of sexuality constructed as and contrained through heterosexuality that the feminist discourse has sometimes entered into a hierarchising of sexualities, suggesting that a different sexuality would enrich women's lives. Rubin (1984) has argued that there is a danger of lesbianism replacing heterosexuality as the correct sexuality. Insofar as it has done so, feminist work, whilst making a radical departure from common sense essentialism, has continued a certain way of speaking about sex. That is, the way forward is still expressed in a certain way of speaking about sexuality and it is still a path that promises to take us toward 'sexual freedom' once one breaks free from 'compulsory heterosexuality'.

It is clear that feminist work has not considered sexuality *per se* as entangling the individual in power/knowledge relations, which was the focus of Foucault's thesis, but has considered, rather, how sexuality has been organised around the one institution of heterosexuality. That is, the *notion* of sexuality has not been the point at which feminism has entered the debate. Rather, feminism has focused on the social *organisation* of sexuality and has not been too concerned with the discursive production of the terms we use to describe sexuality, often using the idea 'sexuality' and the categories of sexuality relatively unproblematically. This is again a matter of how far one takes 'social constructionism'. Feminism has looked at how ideas about sexuality have been socially organised, but Foucault's focus was on the very idea of sexuality that those social organisations brought into usage.

There are therefore a number of points upon which feminist and Foucault's work would deviate from one another. However, there has also been considerable attention paid in the feminist work to the pervasive power of scientific knowledges and to 'pastoral practices', particularly those of the law, which have surrounded sexuality. In this, it seems there is an important convergence with Foucault, one which offers a direction for a feminist utilisation of Foucault.

Questions about how Foucault's work challenges or disrupts feminist work on sexuality have been raised before now. In their introduction to the feminist anthology of work, *Desire: The Politics of Sexuality* (1984), Snitow *et al.* suggest that Foucault's proposal that efforts toward 'sexual freedom' can themselves be traversed by the operations of power is an important contribution to the field. But, they suggest, feminists still need to strive toward sexual freedom since the 'experts' have reigned too long for the feminist discussions of female sexuality to close before they have hardly begun. This would be

> to leave those speakers once again beyond consideration, except insofar as those who previously monopolised the discourse deigned to describe them.
>
> (1983: 2)

The question is how exactly does the feminist work contribute to the discourse of sexuality? Foucault's work causes us to pause and consider feminist work not just as a critique of the ways in which sexuality is spoken about, but also as itself a part of the discourse on sexuality. That is, feminist voices have become themselves powerful and productive within a power/knowledge network.

The feminist 'concern' with sexuality is thus located by Foucault not as a radical shift in our culture but as a continuation of a longstanding concern with sexual practices. Feminist work on incest, as a case in point, might present a break in sociological work, but it may simultaneously be a continuation of a concern with the sexual practices within the family that has been a priority of welfarist and charity discourses and practices up until now. How does feminism continue or subvert ways of speaking about sexuality in that context? Foucault forces one to reflect upon feminist categories and discursive strategies; how do they correspond to other ways of talking about sex? His work cannot be read as prescriptive, as a manual for the 'right' way to speak about sex: rather, it suggests that we engage in a continual questioning of the implications and discursive effects of feminist work. As Sawicki has noted:

> Foucauldian discourse is radical not because it gets at the roots of domination, but inasmuch as it introduces radically new questions and problems concerning prevailing ways of understanding ourselves which continue to dominate our thinking about radical social transformation.
>
> (1988: 176)

For feminism, the radical transformation desired is one which elevates the position of women in society. Here we encounter the single most striking difference between Foucault's thesis in *THS* and feminist work on sexuality. Foucault's central interest is with the production of the concept of sexuality and categories of sexuality ('homosexual', 'heterosexual', 'paedophiliac', etc.) through power/knowledge networks. By contrast, feminists are more interested in those knowledges which create a differential relationship between men and women, or that act against women as a group. Knowledges which suggest that women need men in order to experience sexual satisfaction, which situate lesbianism as a deviant sexual choice, which depict masculine sexuality as inherently predatory, have been considered by feminists not simply as powerful knowledges that constrain all individuals, but as powerful knowledges that differentially constrain women. Crucially, the central concern of feminism is the way in which these ways of understanding sexuality have operated to make women subordinate to men as individuals and as a group.

The major feminist criticism of Foucault's thesis on sexuality

26

therefore is that he fails to consider what one might term the *gendering* aspects of sexuality. This is not the same as the criticism that Foucault 'leaves out' or ignores gender issues, one which has sometimes been levelled at him. Diamond and Quinby, for example, refer to 'gaps' in Foucault's thesis (1988: xv). Yet insofar as Foucault talks about women as a target of the strategies of sexuality, women as embroiled in the process of the deployment of sexuality (e.g. as mothers in the strategy aimed at children and heterosexuality as the 'silent norm'), he is necessarily talking about the creation of gender. What he fails to do is to consider how the strategies of sexuality affect the relationship *between* men and women as gendered individuals. This is the most important aspect of the feminist critique of Foucault's work, the real stumbling block to a Foucauldian feminism.

THS displays a lack of interest in gender not by ignoring gender *per se*, but insofar as it does not consider how the deployment of sexuality has affected the relations between men and women. It is almost as if Foucault depicts individuals in relation to discourses but not in relation to each other; the interaction between people in bed, in sexual abuse, on the street, does not seem to be there. But this is of course a nonsensical statement, since discourses and power relations only exist where there are people and practices which sustain them, and Foucault (the Foucault of *THS* at least) would be the first to agree. One wonders whether this is really about the 'level' of analysis: Foucault does not write about people's lives, their desires nor their abuses in close detail because his concern is with the 'wider' strategies in which they are enveloped. For feminism, therefore, the task is to consider how the knowledges of sexuality impact and intervene with the ways in which gender is understood and lived out, for whilst the relations between men and women are *the* focus of feminism, almost by definition, the construction of other relations will always weave amongst gender relations.

But is my suspicion that gender is a stumbling block not so much because Foucault's concept of sexuality evades gender, but because his concept of *power* seems to preclude a model in which power consistently operates against one group (such as women). It is in their respective conceptions of power that there is a fundamental discord between Foucault and feminism. The problem is both in the notion of the *consistency* of power's operations and, as some feminists have argued (although I would suggest this was not a discussion central to Foucault's work) in the very notion of 'women' as a group which feminism identifies as 'powerless'. Who is included in the group 'women' – how do we identify them? Are women created through discourse in the same way that, for example, 'homosexuals' are? In the next section, therefore, I will investigate the relationship between Foucault and feminism on the question of power. The question of the status of the category 'women' I will reserve until the third section.

POWER

Power is a central theoretical concept in feminism. But feminist work tends to be *about* power rather than a theoretical analysis of how the concept is being used: there has not been much emphasis on developing a 'feminist theory of power' as such. This is partly due to the nature of the feminist task. There are so many areas in which to demonstrate the operations of power that not much time has been spent musing on the concept itself. What counts as power, and how to define power, have not been questions that feminism has spent time debating. It is also partly due to the slippery nature of the concept itself. Discussions within mainstream social theory have become more and more detailed and mathematical in attempting to pin 'power' down. In attempting to answer the question 'what are we interested in when we are interested in power?', Lukes has concluded: 'there are various answers, all deeply familiar . . . yet every attempt at a single general answer to the question has failed and seems likely to fail' (1986: 17). It is possible to make only the most general statement about feminist use of the concept of power. Feminism uses power to refer to exploitation and control. For feminist theory, as for all social theory, this is what power is generally 'about' (Lukes, 1986). In *THS*, Foucault is explicitly concerned with developing a general theory or 'analytics' of power (see especially 1981: 81–102). Addressing the question head on, he details how he understands power to operate both within and beyond the realm of sexuality. In this section I will present Foucault's arguments and explore their implications for feminism.

In *THS* Foucault's remarks are aimed at what he considered the predominant ways of thinking about power at the time of writing. (It is worth noting immediately that feminism was not one of the targets of his accounts, although it has aspects in common with the model he delineates.) Foucault argues that political theory has yet to 'cut off the head of the king' (1981: 88–9), insofar as theorists continue to use a model of power premised on the notion of sovereignty, a conception he terms 'juridico-discursive'. This model characterises power as the word of the sovereign: power lays down the law. 'It speaks, and that is the rule' (1981: 83). In essence, this model of power regards power's operation as the creation of rules or laws whose transgressors will be punished. The conception of power as juridico-discursive is found in twentieth-century analyses of sexuality (such as Marcuse, 1956, and Reich, 1975) which look toward a liberation from the repression of sexuality. Furthermore, this understanding of power is invoked all around us; it is a way of speaking about power that is 'deeply rooted' in the history of the West (1981: 83). Since the Middle Ages, Foucault contends, theorising power has been constrained within such an imagery and language of law.[3]

Foucault argues that power is repeatedly represented in a way that is no longer appropriate: 'the representation of power has remained under the spell of the monarchy' (1981: 88). The judicial monarchy was once characteristic of our societies, but this form of power was 'transitory',

> for while many of its forms have persisted to the present, it has gradually been penetrated by quite new mechanisms of power that are probably irreducible to the representation of law.
>
> (1981: 89)

The important elements of the juridical conception, and Foucault's objections to them, can be summarised as follows:

1 Power operates only in negative ways. In the case of sex and pleasure, 'power can "do" nothing but say no to them' (1981: 83). It acts only by prohibition – 'thou shalt not' – with the prohibition backed up by the threat of punishment. The only effect this power would have is obedience. To this Foucault contrasts the productivity of power.

> Power would be a fragile thing if its only function were to repress, if it worked only through the mode of censorship,

29

exclusion blockage and repression . . . exercising itself only
in a negative way.

(1980a: 59)

2   A binary system is set up by the rule demarcating the licit and
illicit: the forbidden side is repressed. Power works by the
'triple injunction', simultaneously stating that the illicit is not
permitted, preventing it from being articulated but also
denying its existence (1981: 84). Foucault argues against this.
According to him, power works not by a binary system, in
which power's efforts are concentrated on attempting to
repress the illicit whilst the licit are ignored, but by a process
of normalisation. Normalisation works not on the illicit side of
a binary division but everywhere, by setting up a norm to
which people must conform, and according to which people
are judged and placed in an array of positions. Thus the
image of the line gives way to that of a circle with the Norm as
the central ideal position to which people are 'pushed'.

3   Power emanates from a central source, in the historical situation
the monarch, or in political theory the state or a group of
people. To this, Foucault argues that power cannot be
theorised as a possession, and thus it cannot be regarded as
always in the hands of one group. Power is rather a 'complex
strategical situation' that is not encapsulated in a binary
division: 'there is no binary and all encompassing opposition
between rulers and ruled at the root of power relations, and
serving as a general matrix' (1981: 94). Thus Foucault attacks
a second binary division which pervades thinking about power.

4   Following on from 3, there is in the juridico-discursive
conception of power the notion that one might theoretically
overcome power and attain freedom. If the source of power
is identifiable and power is a possession of those identified as
powerful, power can be located and taken away from the
powerful by the powerless. Foucault's disagreement with this
notion of power is based on the argument that one cannot
locate and act upon power in this way because power is all
around us: it is 'omnipresent'. Foucault argues that power is
more complex and elusive than this perspective suggests.

Moving away from the juridical conception of power, Foucault
suggests that the 'little question' of 'what happens?' (1986b: 217)
is the best question by which to approach the study of power

because it avoids assuming any model of power at the outset. Indeed, he suggests that it implicitly poses the possibility that power does not exist, and thereby forces one to seek out and study the actual operations of power. In Foucault's 'analytics'[4] of power, the operation of power has to be studied from 'below', in an ascending analysis (1980a: 99). Confrontations and patterns formed at the local level should be the starting point for a study of power's operations. The focus of a study of power should be the 'concrete but changing soil', the tactics upon which the larger strategies of power are grounded (1980a: 186). In *THS* Foucault speaks of a 'network of power relations' that forms a 'dense web that passes through apparatuses and institutions, without being localised within them' (1981: 96). Power is to be understood, then, 'in the first instance', as

> the multiplicity of force relations immanent in the sphere in which they operate and which constitute their own organisation; as the process which, through ceaseless struggles and confrontations, transforms, strengthens, or reverses them; as the support which these force relations find in one another, thus forming a chain or a system, or, on the contrary, the disjunctions and contradictions which isolate them one from one another; and lastly, as the strategies in which they take effect, whose general design or institutional crystallisation is embodied in the state apparatus, in the formation of law, in the various social hegemonies.
>
> (1981: 92–3)

For Foucault, therefore, the locus of power is dispersed. The state, for example, can only operate on the basis of power relations that exist within the social field, the 'polymorphous techniques of power' (1981: 11). For the theorist, the prescription is not to formulate 'global systematic theory . . . but to analyse the specificity of mechanisms of power, to locate the connections and extensions' (1981: 145). It is these local tactics that work to support what may have appeared at first to be the source of power (1980a: 159). Thus one can speak of strategies of power only once one has traced the 'tactics', the micro-techniques of power.[5] This also means that whilst the aims and logic of strategies of power may be clear, there is no one who can be said to have invented them, and few to have formulated them. Power does not necessarily reside with those who make decisions:

[Power relations are] great anonymous, almost unspoken strategies which coordinate the loquacious tactics whose 'inventors' or decisionmakers are often without hypocrisy.

(1981: 95)

Furthermore, Foucault argues that where power operates there is resistance. He is making a point about the necessity of power. If there were no resistance, there would be no need for power's operations. Thus resistance is not outside power, working against power from without but, Foucault insists, is in relation with power. The point is not that there is no escaping power, but that there are a 'multiplicity of points of resistance' that exist in the strategic power network (1981: 95–6). Resistances to power can be different in character. They may be progressive or conservative. There are some that are 'possible, necessary, improbable; others that are spontaneous, savage, solitary, concerted, rampant or violent; still others that are quick to compromise, interested or sacrificial' (1981: 96). Occasionally, Foucault concedes, there may be 'massive binary divisions' between those who resist and the operation of power, but, he argues,

> more often one is dealing with mobile and transitory points of resistance, producing cleavages in a society that shift about, fracturing unities and effecting regroupings, furrowing across individuals themselves, cutting them up and remoulding them, marking off irreducible regions in them, in their bodies and minds.

(1981: 96)

In stressing the role of resistance, Foucault is also making an important contrast between violence, where the possibility of resistance is taken away, and power, the exercise of which is necessary only when there is the possibility of the 'targets' resisting (see, e.g., 1988: 123). Power operates not to stop its targets acting, but to control their actions:

> what defines a relationship of power is that it is a mode of action which does not act directly and immediately on others. Instead it *acts upon their actions*: an action on an action, on existing actions or on those which may arise in the present or the future. A relationship of violence acts upon a body or upon things; it forces, it bends, . . . it

destroys, or it closes the door on all possibilities. . . . On the other hand a power relationship can only be articulated on the basis of two elements which are each indispensable if it is really to be a power relationship: that 'the other' (the one over whom power is exercised) be thoroughly recognised and maintained to the very end as a person who acts; and that, faced with a relationship of power, a whole field of responses, reactions, results and possible inventions may open up.

(1982: 220; emphasis added)

The operation of power can achieve aims much more smoothly and successfully than the imposition of violence. As well as the economic cost of violence, there is a 'specifically political cost': 'If you are too violent, you risk provoking revolts' (1980a: 155). The sorts of powers Foucault saw in operation involved much quieter, more subtle tactics.

Foucault's general comments on power are fleshed out toward the end of *THS* with the conception of power to which he gives the name 'bio-power'. This is a power over life. In contrast with the power of the sovereign which was the right to decide whether to 'take life or let live', a right of seizure that included ultimately the lives of the people, this newer power exercises power over life through various tactics that incite, reinforce, control, monitor and organise people's lives, so that 'one might say that the ancient right to *take* life or *let* live was replaced by a power to *foster* life or *disallow* it to the point of death' (1981: 138; original emphasis).

There are two poles to bio-power. One of these poles centres on 'the body as a machine' (1981: 139). Although he does not state it, Foucault is referring back to his previous work, *Discipline and Punish* (1979a), in which he provides a detailed exposition of disciplinary power and its operations on the body. In *THS* it is summarised thus:

[The body's] disciplining, the optimisation of its capabilities, the extortion of its forces, the parallel increase of its usefulness and its docility, its integration into systems of efficient and economic controls, all this was ensured by the procedures of power that characterised the *disciplines: an anatomo-politics of the human body.*

(1981: 139)

Discipline is a power which works through the 'meticulous control of the operations of the body' (1979a: 137). Its effect is 'subjected and practised bodies, "docile" bodies' (1979a: 138): discipline 'increases the forces of the body (in economic terms of utility) and diminishes those same forces (in political terms of obedience)' (1979a: 138). Discipline operates through techniques which: order space, separating individuals from one another; control activity, imposing timetables that disallow idleness, enforcing specific and detailed postures on the 'inmate' population; organise the passing of time into successive stages through which individuals progress; and compose the forces of bodies as an efficient organisation in order to obtain some specific result, be it economic or otherwise (1979a: 141–69). Foucault traces the operations of discipline within institutions such as the prison, schools, the military, factories. Techniques of disciplinary power were often ones that had been in use in monastic institutions, but in the seventeenth and eighteenth centuries, Foucault argues, they spread to several institutions, and from there to other areas of society, creating 'what might be called in general the disciplinary society' (1979a: 209).[6]

Foucault describes the three methods of disciplinary power. First, discipline operates by hierarchical observation, which makes it possible for a single gaze to see everything. Foucault argues that disciplinary power utilises the observation powers of the Panopticon, Jeremy Bentham's architectural design published at the end of the eighteenth century.[7] The organisation of the Panopticon made it possible to observe without being seen, such that the individuals had always to act as though they were being watched. The result is the 'automatic functioning of power'. This is how the Panopticon works:

[A]t the periphery an annular building; at its centre a tower; this tower is pierced with wide windows that open onto the inner side of the ring; the peripheric building is divided into cells, each of which extends the width of the building; they have two windows, one on the inside, corresponding to the windows of the tower; the other, on the outside, allows the light to cross the cell from one end to the other. All that is needed, then, is to place a supervisor in a central tower and to shut up in each cell a madman, a patient, a condemned man, a worker or a schoolboy. By the effect of backlighting, one can observe from the tower, standing out precisely against the light, the small captive shadows in the cells of the periphery . . . [they are] perfectly individualised and constantly visible. . . . Visibility is a trap.

(1979a: 200)

Secondly, discipline involves normalising judgement, mentioned above, which compares individuals and differentiates between them according to a desired norm. This normalisation produces homogeneity by measuring all individuals against the same 'norm', but at the same time it individualises, measuring and differentiating between each and every one. The third method is the examination, which combines both hierarchical observation and normalising judgement. Through the examination individuals are classified and, if considered necessary, punished through the penal system at the heart of disciplinary institutions. Through disciplinary techniques, an individual becomes a 'case', as a knowledge of him or her is built up. This is a 'reversal of the political axis of individualisation' (1979a: 192). In societies past, it was the sovereign and the rich who were marked as individuals, in the sense of rare personages, 'by rituals, written accounts or visual reproduction' (1979: 192); with disciplinary power it is rather those at the other end of the axis who are 'individualised':

[B]y surveillance rather than ceremonies, by observation rather than commemorative accounts, by comparative measures that have the 'norm' as their reference rather than genealogies giving ancestors as points of reference; by 'gaps' rather than by deeds.

(1979a: 193)

It is with reference to disciplinary power that Foucault most clearly makes the argument that power is productive. Disciplinary mechanisms are not repressive, exclusionary techniques that mask and conceal, but are *productive* techniques. Power is productive in the sense of producing the bodily movements that it dictates, and any economic results in which these movements result. But more profoundly, power is productive in the sense of 'producing domains of objects and rituals of truth', knowledges and the 'individuals' that are known through those knowledges (1979a: 194).

35

The second pole of bio-power, to which the first is connected by 'a whole intermediary cluster of relations' (1981: 139), is directed toward the 'species body' as a whole. The target of this power is the life of the population: 'propagation, births and mortality, the level of health, life expectancy and longevity, with all the conditions that can cause these to vary' (1981: 139). These were supervised and regulated. Statistics began to be collected, housing was inspected and the movement of the population monitored. Thus demography emerged as a discipline, with predictions relating population growth to wealth, resources to migration (1981: 141). The interconnections between the two poles of bio-power (equivalent, it seems, to tactics and strategies) are joined by concrete arrangements. An example of the ways in which the two poles of bio-power interconnect is that of family planning. The regulation of the population described by Foucault as the strategy directed at the 'Malthusian couple' relied upon the operations of disciplinary power at the individual level. Family planning requires individuals to organise their sexual activity: it is a control of activity, timing, movements. This is a form of discipline that allows the incitement or restriction of procreation at the 'population' level. One might speculate, furthermore, on how the other strategies of the deployment of sexuality involve both poles of bio-power, although Foucault himself discusses none of these. One might argue, for example, that the strategy of particular relevance to this book, the pedagogisation of children's sex, involves the organisation of space in the household as children are kept separate from one another and from parental sexual activity, thereby instituting the parental (and other) gaze over the children's bodies, whilst the dangers of masturbation for the race as a whole were expounded, justifying and encouraging this disciplinary power around children in the home in terms of the population.

The deployment of sexuality was, Foucault suggests, one of the most important of the bio-political apparatuses. It seems to be more than an example of power for Foucault. Its importance lies in the fact that sex is the link between the two poles of bio-power, at the 'juncture between the "body" and the "population" ', so that it 'became a crucial target of a power organised around the management of life rather than the menace of death' (1981: 147).

Foucault's work on power: the implications for feminism

There is a broad similarity between Foucault's point of departure and that of feminist analyses in that they both reject the same models of power. Feminism, too, has been critical of liberal theory and of Marxism (Hartmann, 1981; Martin, 1988). The feminist dissatisfaction with liberalism and Marxism, however, is based on a different charge from Foucault's dissatisfaction, namely the absence of women in the traditional analyses. But feminists have been more willing than Foucault to explore these models, spawning several different revisions (Walby, 1986). The dissatisfaction, then, is a similar point of departure, but this similarity does not run very far. Nevertheless, an important component of the rejection that both feminism and Foucault have in common is that the traditional liberal and Marxist often uphold a public/private dichotomy, missing the point that the operation of power is just as central in the 'private' areas of life, concerning 'our bodies, our day to day existences' (Foucault, 1980a: 187). Similarly, so-called 'second wave' feminism criticised the sexual liberation movement of the 1960s and 1970s for failing to analyse the political dimension of sexual relations (Shulman, 1980). Feminists have argued, as does Foucault, against the idea that there has been 'sexual liberation', pointing out that a freedom to engage in sexual relations does not mean the erasure of power relations in the realm of sexuality.

Some of the most convincing feminist work using Foucault's writings on power has focused on his notion of disciplinary power. Foucault's detailed work on the operations of disciplinary power on the body have been applied to the study of the construction of femininity.[8] Sandra Lee Bartky (1988) uses Foucault's exposition of disciplinary power in an analysis of the ways in which women's bodies are disciplined in the name of femininity. She states:

> Foucault treats the body throughout as if it were one, as if the bodily experiences of men and women did not differ and as if men and women bore the same relationship to the characteristic institutions of modern life . . . he is blind to those disciplines that produce a modality of embodiment that is peculiarly feminine.
>
> (1988: 63–4)

Bartky applies Foucault's ideas persuasively to an examination of the different ways in which women's bodies are 'rendered docile' through the disciplinary practices of exercise and diet, of correct body language, and of fashion and make-up. In particular Bartky draws upon Foucault's analysis of the normalising power effects of the Panopticon. In this trap of visibility, power is both visible and unverifiable for the inmate. It is visible due to the presence of the observation tower constantly before him or her. Yet it is unverifiable because the inmate can never know whether s/he is being watched at any particular moment (Foucault, 1979a: 201). One of the prime effects of disciplinary power, due to the fact that the visible individual can never know whether he or she is being watched, is the 'automatic' functioning of power. The inmates watch over themselves:

> He who is subjected to a field of visibility and who knows it assumes responsibility for the constraints of power; he makes them play spontaneously upon himself; he inscribes in himself the power relation in which he simultaneously plays both roles; he becomes the principle of his own subjection.
>
> (Foucault, 1979a: 202–3)

Bartky sees in Foucault's work an analytic framework by which to elucidate the practice of femininity. She states: 'Woman lives her body as seen by another, by an anonymous patriarchal Other' (1988: 72). Bartky considers the various ways in which women's bodies are manipulated by the demands of contemporary society. Women are encouraged to judge themselves through bodily appearance and movements, and to use their bodies to display the signs of femininity. Bartky argues that this is not just a case of women being marked differently from men. There is a value judgement being placed upon women. They are marked not simply as different but as inferior:

> Are we dealing in all this merely with sexual difference? Scarcely. The disciplinary practices I have described are part of the process by which the ideal body of femininity – and hence the feminine body-subject – is constructed; in doing this, they produce a 'practiced and subjected' body, that is, a body on which an inferior status has been inscribed.
>
> (1988: 71)

38

This is the mode in which it has been argued feminists should use Foucault's work on power. That is, not to seek the 'origin of tyranny' but to examine 'the interactions and the histories of daily occurrences that sustain systems of normalisation and control' (McWhorter, 1986). Instead of searching 'backwards' for an answer to women's subordination, feminists should concentrate on the ways in which women are kept subordinate to men through the operations of these subtle techniques.

However, there are problems with a feminist/Foucauldian meeting relating to the notion of power. These arise because of Foucault's rejection of juridico-discursive power, for this is the model of power that is implicit in much feminist work. In particular, the ruler/ruled division of the juridico-discursive power might be seen to be replicated in feminist analyses to the extent that men are theorised as having power over women. To draw this out a little, feminism might be seen to use the juridico-discursive model to the extent that:

1 it depicts a *hierarchical* binary division with men 'on top';
2 it depicts men as *possessing* power;
3 it depicts this as a *static* power relation.

As will be recalled, for Foucault power is not something that can be possessed, but exists only in its exercise, and since that exercise takes place all around us, it is inaccurate to posit at the outset a great binary division in power. The overall sense that Foucault's work gives of power is as fluid and unpredictable. Power is much more mobile and unstable than the binary division contained within juridico-discursive models of power suggests. For feminism, however, the argument that power is structured along lines of gender has been a fundamental point of departure.

Nancy Hartsock has argued that Foucault's model of power cannot capture the domination of women by men that feminist work addresses and reveals. Writing from a 'materialist' feminist perspective, she considers the lack of a sense of social structures in Foucault's work both an inadequacy of his theory and an indicator of the dangers that a Foucauldian feminism faces. She has argued:

> [H]is stress on heterogeneity and the specificity of each situation leads him to lose track of social structures and

instead to focus on how individuals experience and exercise power. Individuals, he argues, 'are always in the position of simultaneously undergoing and exercising this power [Foucault, 1980a: 197].' . . . With this move Foucault has made it very difficult to locate domination, including domination in gender relations.

(1990: 169)

By retaining the term 'domination', Hartsock seems to wish to hold on to aspects of the model of power outlined in the three points above. Seeing the potential clash between feminism and Foucault, Hartsock's resolution is to dismiss the Foucauldian model of power. However, her hostility to Foucault stems from an established belief about the existence of domination, and her rejection is argued on pragmatic grounds. That is, the rejection is made not through the argument that we *need* to locate domination. Hartsock does not take on the challenge of Foucault's analytics of power because she establishes her position without considering whether one *can* simply talk about domination as always already there. Other feminist writers have also noted the tension around the issue of power but resolved it differently. Phelan (1990) uses Foucault to argue that feminist writers such as Rich (1980) and Daly (1978) are misguided to depict men as statically holding power over women. Phelan's reading of Foucault is a sympathetic one, one that allows his 'analytics' of power to reach feminist conclusions:

Foucault's work should lead us to suspect that these various sites of oppression are indeed various, that we must examine them in their particularity, as operations that may oppose and challenge one another even as they tend toward a common end for women . . . unity is a production, shifting and unstable, as are divisions.

(1990: 428)

Phelan's conclusion is appealing because it allows for the complexities of power's operations without abandoning the feminist argument that in some broad way women share a common oppression. It refuses to allow women to be painted as merely the victims of male domination, a depiction that has been criticised within feminism, by emphasising the power that women exercise in spheres where they do have the opportunity to be powerful, or in direct resistance to the exercise of male power (this later type of resistance has been highlighted in recent feminist analyses of male violence; see Kelly, 1988b, and Gordon, 1986; 1988). *Contra* Hartsock, therefore, much feminist work now argues against a simple powerful/powerless division. Thus Foucault and feminist thought move somewhat closer together.

However, such a perspective means that the patterns that feminists have pointed to, the shifting unity of repeated discrimination, appear as mere coincidences in Foucault's model of power. Although Foucault's work is useful to feminism in thinking through the contingency of power relations, feminism needs to be able to name the familiar patterns that emerge. Thus feminists might make the distinction between the operations of power and *domination* as a name given to a state of 'perpetual asymmetry', a distinction that Foucault himself conceded in a late interview. Foucault explained (using the example of husband and wife, interestingly) that domination is where

> the relations of power are fixed in such a way that they are perpetually asymmetrical and the margin of liberty is extremely limited. To take an example, very paradigmatic to be sure: in the traditional conjugal relation of the eighteenth and nineteenth centuries, we cannot say that there was only male power: the woman herself could do a lot of things: be unfaithful to him, extract money from him, refuse him sexually. She was, however, subject to a state of domination, in the measure where all that was finally no more than a certain number of tricks which never brought about a reversal of the situation.
>
> (In Bernauer and Rasmussen, 1988: 12)

Thus domination is a situation, still based on the operations of unstable tactics of power, but where a reversal in power relations appears to be almost impossible. For feminism, domination would denote the patterns of asymmetry between men and women that repeatedly emerge from feminist investigations. But such a Foucauldian/feminist perspective retains an awareness of contradictions within that 'domination' as well as an optimism, because if power is exercised not possessed, contingent rather than static, feminist opposition to the various operations of power may expect to identify more gaps and weaknesses in power's operations.

41

Referring back to the three aspects of power at which a feminist/Foucault meeting may become difficult, therefore, it can be argued that the first of the three (hierarchy) can be retained even as the other two points (the ability to possess power and the static nature of power relations) are relinquished. Foucault's argument that the binary model of power which depicts power as a possession and as static captures neither the contingency of power nor the fact that power is always an exercise is convincing and illuminating. For feminism, there has already been a general move toward acknowledging the complexities and contradictions in power's operations (and in the body of 'women' of which feminism speaks). However, feminist analyses are about the demonstration of hierarchy. It is this hierarchy that Foucault seems to concede with the label 'domination'. Domination, in a feminist use of Foucault, would be the 'perpetual asymmetry' between men and women in the exercise and the effects of power's operations. Thus although men cannot be said to possess power, nor to exclusively exercise power, feminist analysis demonstrates the differential and hierarchical positions of men and women in relations which repeatedly accord men the greater access to the exercise of power.

DISCOURSE, POWER/KNOWLEDGE, TRUTH AND POLITICS

The definition of discourse is no simple matter. For Foucault, it is both less and more than 'language'. It is less in that discourse is not a description of the whole language system, it is not concerned with Saussure's 'langue'. It is more in that it is not just speaking and writing, but entails social and political relations: one cannot dissociate discourse from a social context where relations of power and knowledge circulate. Although he treats it differently at different times, the importance of discourse runs throughout Foucault's work. Foucault addresses the concept of discourse most explicitly in *The Archaeology of Knowledge* (1972), where he is interested in developing a theory of discourses and a methodology for studying them, which he termed 'archaeology'. Archaeology is an historical method which is essentially a rewriting, a systematic description of a discourse object (1972: 140). It considers the formation of specific knowledges without translating the project into a discussion of the individuals who

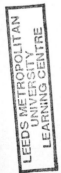

hold that knowledge: its focus is on the rules of formation of knowledges, rules defining objects, techniques and processes of validating knowledge. His concern at this time was with the identification of rules that govern 'discursive formations' unknown to the speakers within them.

Foucault describes his project in *The Archaeology of Knowledge* as an attempt to show that

> to speak is to do something – something other than to express what one thinks, to translate what one knows . . . to show that to add a statement to a pre-existing series of statements is to perform a complicated and costly gesture, which involves conditions (and not only a situation, a context and motives) and rules (not the logical and linguistic rules of construction); to show that a change in the order of discourse does not presuppose 'new ideas', a little invention and creativity, a different mentality, but transformations in practice, perhaps also in neighbouring practices, and in their common articulation.
>
> (1972: 209)

Foucault's interest in *The Archaeology of Knowledge* was in what Dreyfus and Rabinow term 'serious speech acts' (1986: 48) and the discursive formations of which these speech acts form a part. The speech acts are serious when they have been validated by some sort of institutionalised test, with some community of experts to justify them as knowledge. The approach is a 'diagnosis' (Foucault, 1972: 206) that looks at the state of discourses and the patterns they form. It seeks out the rules that place some form of constraint on what the speakers can say. It is an approach that does not concern itself with the truth of what is said but is more in the descriptive mode (1972: 27), attentive to changes in discourses and the timing of statements:

> The analysis of statements then is a historical analysis but one that avoids all interpretation: it does not question things said as to what they were hiding, what they were really saying, in spite of themselves, the unspoken element they contain . . . but on the contrary, it questions them as to their mode of existence . . . what it means for them to have appeared when they did, they and no others.
>
> (1972: 109)

By the time Foucault wrote *THS*, his concerns were less with the search for rules, regularities and the formation of discourses and more with questions of the relationships between power, knowledge and discourse.[9] During the period between *The Archaeology of Knowledge* and *THS*, Foucault's own understanding of what he was doing altered. Whilst it still contained important aspects of archaeology, the later approach, which he named 'genealogy', resulted from important changes in his understanding of his work. The interest Foucault had had in the rules which governed discourses disappears, and, although discourses are still the object of study and the level at which Foucault's analysis 'enters', the abstract and generalised approach to discourse of *The Archaeology of Knowledge* is replaced by a more 'grounded' interest in the ways that discourse is both built upon networks of power/knowledge and produces certain power effects.

'Power/knowledge' refers to the processes by which power and knowledge interact. The interactions may be complex and contradictory; it is the genealogist's job to study these interactions, the processes whereby, through the operations of power, knowledges are formed, the implications of the implementation of knowledge claims, and so on. Foucault does not argue that power and knowledge are the same thing. Rather, they are entwined:

> [If] I had said, or meant, that knowledge was power, I would have said so, and, having said so, I would have had nothing more to say, since, having made them identical, I don't see why I would have taken the trouble to show the different relations between them.
>
> (1988: 264)

Sometimes Foucault speaks of power as if it were *always* entwined with knowledge:

> [P]ower produces knowledge (and not simply by encouraging it because it serves power or applying it because it is useful) . . . power and knowledge directly imply one another . . . there is no power relation without the correlative constitution of a field of knowledge, nor any knowledge that does not presuppose and constitute at the same time power relations.
>
> (1979a: 27)

In his later interviews, however, Foucault argues that it is not the case that all knowledges are the result of or continue power relations. He suggests in an interview that his analysis of the relations between power and knowledge concern human sciences, and do not concern the 'exact sciences'[10] at all (1988: 106). He also states that it is possible to find knowledges of the human sciences that are 'independent' of power (1988: 106). Thus one cannot make broad claims about all knowledge and power: it is in the detailed study of specific areas that one illuminates any interconnections between power and knowledge. Thus genealogy is the study of the concrete and disparate arrangements upon which knowledges and their respective 'objects' have been constructed and the power relations that are there deployed. Foucault's concern is with how discourses, and their truth effects, that is, the ways in which they are acted upon and towards as True, are maintained by and function to uphold, to resist or to alter relations of power.[11]

In *The Archaeology of Knowledge*, Foucault had argued that discourses, as opposed to being simply signs that refer to or represent some reality, are

> practices that systematically form the object of which they speak. Of course discourses are composed of signs; but what they do is more than use these signs to designate things. It is this *more* that renders them irreducible to the language (langue) and to speech. It is this 'more' that we must reveal and describe.
>
> (1972: 49)

Arguably this investigation of the 'more than speech' is still Foucault's project in *THS* insofar as he interrogates genealogically the various discourses on sexuality for the way they have created the objects of which they speak, such as the natural but dangerous sexuality of children, homosexuality, hysterical female sexuality or 'normal' responsible procreative sexuality, or the more general object 'sexuality' created through the combination of these. The 'more than speech' is still Foucault's terrain since it corresponds to what he describes in *THS* as the power/knowledge network that constitutes 'the deployment of sexuality'.

Genealogy is an historical method, interrogating current discourses in search of their place within historical contingencies, but it is a method opposed to traditional history. It does not seek to record the progress and continuity of societies. It avoids the search for depth, avoids the search for what 'really happened' underneath historical events, and locates its analysis instead on the surface, on the details; it is 'meticulous and patiently documentary' (1986a: 76). The notion that there is a deep and true meaning of history is relocated as a function of the historical discourses that claim as much. Genealogy is opposed to the totalising effects of 'superhistories' such as Hegelian or Marxian histories that see one great plan unfolding as time progresses. Foucault wants to offer an analysis that illuminates specific aspects of present society, specific present discourses, by tracing their history and that history's interconnections with strategies of power and knowledge in their peculiarity.

This approach to history is what Foucault terms a 'history of the present' (1979a: 31). It has an 'unabashed contemporary orientation' (Dreyfus and Rabinow, 1986: 119), in the sense that it begins with a self-reflective diagnosis of the present. In *THS*, for example, Foucault points to the way we currently (in the 1970s at least) speak of sexuality. In particular, he considers the way that speaking about sex, confessing our sexual deeds and desires is considered a path to true and deep understanding of our selves. The historian of the present then considers where such a way of talking arose, how it has been changed, shaped through time by forces of power and knowledge, not in order to discover the origins, the moment at which one can argue it began, but to follow 'the complex course', to 'identify the accidents, the minute derivations or conversely, the complete reversals . . . that gave birth to those things that continue to exist and have value for us' (1986a: 81).

Foucault described himself as an 'empiricist' (1988: 106); that is, he wanted to provide the detailed evidence for his assertions. Thus, although Foucault's position does seem to be that which he stated in 1967: 'There is nothing absolutely primary to interpret because, when all is said and done, underneath it all everything is already interpretation' (quoted in Dreyfus and Rabinow, 1986: 107), it is not the case that any reading of history will do. Foucault would argue, to stick with an example from *THS*, that this *is*, in terms of the evidence available to him, how the current discourse on sexuality is historically linked to the confession. He claims to trace the confession and its links to power as they have really

46

occurred. Foucault then locates this specific trace (of the confession) within the more general power strategy, the deployment of sexuality. Thus Foucault stated: 'I am fully aware that I have never written anything other than fictions.... I would not say that they were outside the truth. It seems plausible to me to make fictions work within truth' (1980a: 193).

There has been opposition to a feminist/Foucauldian meeting that has focused on his arguments around discourse. Foucault's arguments have been grouped (perhaps hastily) with writers generally referred to as 'postmodern', and the general epistemological argument that there are only ever truths of the world, never a Truth to be discovered. The possible antithesis here concerns the relationship of his theoretical stance to feminist political practice. To break this down a little, the problem is that Foucault's work is seen to represent a challenge to feminist epistemology, that is, to feminist claims to Truth, and consequently to feminist politics.

The problem Foucault's position holds for feminism has been interpreted as follows:

> [Feminism has been] based on the premiss that *we as feminists can speak authentically, can speak the truth* of ourselves for all women by virtue of our supposed exclusion from male culture and as a result of our rejection of their meanings. The tendency to place women outside culture, to define femininity in terms of an absolute exclusion and consequent innocence with respect to language and ideology ... [assumes] that we can shed what is supposedly a false consciousness imposed and maintained from outside.
>
> (Martin, 1988: 15; emphasis added)

Read from within Foucault's framework, the claim that feminism has access to the Truth becomes problematic, for it amounts to the claim that feminists are unaffected by the various discourses which construct our perceptions of Truth. Hence the concern is that by refusing to privilege any one discourse (such as the feminist) above another, Foucault's analysis disallows feminism the ability to enter political argument about sex-oppression (this is the worry of Balbus, 1982, for example).

Foucault's various comments on truth are somewhat confusing, especially where he makes broad and almost rhetorical generalisations about his own position. For example, where he argues that 'we are forced to produce the truth of power that our society demands, of which it has a need in order to function' (1980a: 93) or that 'each society has its own regime of truth, its general politics of truth: that is, the type of discourse which it accepts and makes function as true' (1980a: 131), it does seem that one is left without being able to claim any statement as true without it being always the result of the operations of a society-wide power. Foucault's arguments are the most persuasive when he is talking about particular discourses and with specific examples.

It was never Foucault's argument that truth does not exist, nor that everything is in people's minds, nor that if power and truth are connected, the truth propounded is automatically false. Foucault's works are better understood as investigations of 'problematisations', which he defined as 'the totality of discursive and non-discursive practices that introduces something into the play of truth and false and constitutes it as an object of thought (whether in the form of moral reflection, scientific knowledge, political analysis, etc.)' (1988: 257). He wanted to 'question over and over again what is postulated as self evident, to disturb people's mental habits' (1988: 265).

Feminists have seen in this sort of approach the opportunity to critique various truths that are propounded about women and gender relations. The task of feminism becomes 'the deconstruction of truth and analysis of the power effects claims to truth entail' (Smart, 1990: 82). This mode of feminist analysis is one that follows Foucault in its disentangling of the power/ knowledge relations that (in)form discourses and the practices based upon them.

> The gaps, silences and ambiguities of discourses provide the possibility for resistance, for a questioning of the dominant discourse, its revision or mutation. Within these silences and gaps new discourses can be formulated that challenge the dominant discourse. This theory of discourse and their mutability provides an accurate understanding of the task of feminism.
>
> (Hekman, 1990: 189–90)

The problem this raises for feminism is that it makes it difficult to answer the question: 'where does feminist discourse come from?' That is, feminists can criticise truth claims, but on what basis? How can feminists claim any authority for their statements?

Feminist claims are often said to derive from thinking about the political dimensions of women's lives 'as women' through meeting in groups to discuss common experiences: 'consciousness-raising'. However, feminists have questioned the validity of consciousness-raising as a method. One major criticism is that when some segment of the female population is not represented, claims to the experience of all women are unrepresentative, and consequently the experience of some women is set up as the experience of all. Although feminism has become more 'theoretically aware' of the differences between women (of age, 'race', able-bodiedness) and the exclusionary claims of some feminist work, this did not lead to an immediate epistemological change in feminism, such as a decision that to make truth claims was impossible. Rather 'the chief imperative was to listen, to become aware of one's biases, prejudices' (Bordo, 1990a: 138), so that there was still a search for true, correct feminist perspectives based on a more representative sample of women.

Within debates on feminist epistemology, 'experience' has been criticised as a suspect basis on which to form feminist theory: 'experience must be the most unreliable source of theoretical production that we could possibly have chosen' (Belsey, quoted in Gunew, 1990: 27). There is a danger that claims made about women will become claims about some essential womanhood, ignoring the social construction of the perception of difference from men (Gunew, 1990). Using experience as the basis of feminist claims implies that women are untouched by the various constructions of Woman (Gunew, 1990), and will be able to stand outside societal constructions that inform perceptions and see the Truth:

> [T]he claim that women will produce an accurate description of reality, either because they are women or because they are more oppressed, appears to be highly implausible. Given the diversity and fallibility of all human knowers, there is no good reason to believe that women are any less prone to error, deception and distortion than men ... [This is] to fail to grasp the manifold ways in which all human experiences ... are mediated by theoretical suppositions embedded in language and culture.
> (Hawkeshead, 1989: 544)

Thus it seems that that whilst the critique of present truths advocated by both Smart (1990) and Hekman (1990) is an attractive strategy for feminists to adopt, there is a stumbling block here, one that concerns all attempts to speak the truth. There is no easy path out of this, but the path left open for feminists is certainly not to stop talking or to renounce any feminist claims. Rather, there is a need to be reflexive about feminism's 'conditions of existence' (Gunew, 1990), the powerful consequences of feminist discourse, its terms and its conclusions: a continual questioning of feminism's 'mental habits'. That is, feminists can see their own claims not as the Truth, but, as Foucault saw his, 'fictions that work within the truth'.

The most radical questioning that has taken place to date has been around the very category 'woman'. This is not just a debate about differences among women, but a debate about the division male/female. If feminist knowledge is about women we have to know who is a woman. There has been some feminist work which has suggested through Foucault that 'women' is a discursive category that can be problematised in much the same way that categories of sexuality can. Judith Butler (1990a) has drawn upon Foucault's *THS* as well as his comments in an introduction to the memoirs of Herculine Barbin, 'a nineteenth-century French hermaphrodite' (1980b), in making her argument that the notion of 'sex' has to be rethought.

In his introduction to the memoirs, Foucault sketches an analysis of the discursive construction of two sexes (1980b: i-xiii). He argues that for a long time hermaphrodites were believed to have two sexes, and there was no suggestion that they had a true underlying sex, either male or female. But biological theories which suggested that sexuality flowed from anatomical sex, judicial conceptions of the individual and the growth of administrative regulation in modern life all led, Foucault suggests, to a rejection of the idea that a body could have two sexes. Thus the doctor became the expert and the task in such cases became the determination of what was hidden beneath the ambiguous appearances of such individuals. Doctors imposed on Barbin's body, Foucault argues, a 'game of truth' (1980b: xiii), and 'in an order of things where one might have imagined that all that counted was the reality of the body and the intensity of its pleasures' (1980b: vii) they demanded that each individual has a true sex which had to be 'obeyed'.

Butler reads Foucault's argument as an illustration of how 'an hermaphroditic or intersexed body implicitly exposes and refutes the regulative strategies of sexual categorisation' (1990a: 96). She outlines the possible antithesis with feminism:

> Where feminism takes the category of sex and, thus, according to [Foucault], the binary restriction on gender, as its point of departure, Foucault understands his own project to be an inquiry into how the category of 'sex' and sexual difference are constructed within discourse as necessary features of bodily identity.
>
> (1990a: 96)

Butler investigates the argument that sex is not a fact of anatomy, but a 'fact' created by discourse: 'Is "the body" or "the sexed body" the firm foundation on which gender and systems of compulsory sexuality operate?' (1990a: 129). Butler argues against the notion that each body has a sex, an underlying force or truth within the body that causes the anatomical shape of the body. This is the 'trope of interiority' (1990a: 134), the notion that anatomy is the sign of (an inner) sex. Where feminists have argued that gender is not within the body but a cultural/discursive phenomenon, Butler argues for a similar move with regard to 'sex'. It is a way of talking about our selves, not an unproblematic 'fact' of anatomy. Butler recognises that Foucault waivers on his arguments about the body, sometimes speaking of the body as if it were a prediscursive materiality (on a couple of occasions in *THS*), but at others as the 'inscribed surface of events' (Foucault, 1977: 148). Nevertheless, she uses his approach to argue that the designation of sex is a discursive operation.

In feminism, Butler suggests, sex is often regarded as the 'hard' fact on which malleable gender constructions work. Her argument is that although obviously preferable to conservative discourses, in which sex is spoken of as the internal cause of one's gender (and, furthermore, of one's sexuality), feminism has not yet done enough deconstructing. Sex, as well as gender, is part of this strategy. Barbin's case, which illustrates the social processes that are set in motion as soon as the anatomy is not easily classified, highlights the fact that male and female are ways of talking about bodies, ways of categorising bodies into two mutually exclusive groups. Once the reality of a hermaphrodite was refused, the question became one of either/or: 'which sex is s/he?' Butler suggests that a similar process continues in contemporary investigations that focus on chromosones and genes rather than anatomy.[12] This argument has been accepted by other feminist writers. Kaplan and Rogers (1990) have argued that the designation of the labels 'male' or 'female' result from a process of decision-making, not a description of 'obvious' facts. There are several different combinations of outward signs, the internal organisation of reproductive organs and chromosonal 'evidence'. Moreover, medical knowledge and common sense can often disagree.

Butler argues that feminism's domain should not be only that of gender production and reproduction, but also that of the designation of sex. Otherwise, feminism becomes 'an analysis which makes that category [sex] presuppositional [and thereby] uncritically extends and further legitimates that regulative strategy as a power/knowledge regime' (1990a: 96).

Butler's arguments[13] point to an antithesis between Foucault and feminism that centres on the status of the term 'sex', meaning the division male/female. Butler's stance is feared by some feminists, who see this move as leaving feminism without a subject ('women'). For example, Linda Alcoff argues that a position in which 'the category "woman" is a fiction' leads only to 'a negative feminism, deconstructing everything and refusing to construct anything' (1988: 417–18). Others have argued for a strategic approach to this tension, suggesting that feminism should engage in

> simultaneously using and questioning the category 'women'. Common sense tells us that it is a real category, so much so that our political agenda must be shaped by it, and yet we may question its history and its use.
>
> (Phelan, 1990: 434)

However, in following this line of argument, it is worth noting a point made by Bordo (1990a), who contends that the refusal to use the category 'women' on grounds of its false inclusivity can become too dogmatic a methodological imperative. She argues that whilst generalisations about gender can obscure and exclude, there 'are dangers in too wholesale a commitment to either dual *or* multiple grids' (1990a: 149). The danger, she claims, is that the deconstruction of 'women' as caused by 'gender scepticism' may lead to the loss of feminism's political force such that the commonalities that women do suffer are left unaddressed. This point is relevant to Butler's form of 'gender scepticism'; the questioning of 'women' may be a useful tool for anti-feminists.

However, the theoretical position Butler espouses need not obscure the subject of feminism even as it is rethought as not straightforwardly 'women' but 'those persons who are labelled as and continually constructed as women'. The notion that we each have a 'sex' located in the body is the foundation of several discourses that work to the detriment of women, ways of speaking which obscure the social discourses that repeatedly attempt to 'pin' people to a sex (and very often, as a result, to a gender and to a sexuality, i.e. heterosexuality). Understanding the ways in which that division is maintained and maintains power relations is the task ahead.

Much of the unease about the 'questioning our truths' position is centred on the practical, political implications of such a stance. Hekman sums up the critique thus:

> Foucault's critics take the position that his approach definitely precludes principled political action because the logic of his analysis denies the possibility of anything but a relative conception of truth.
>
> (1990: 175)

Foucault's positions on truth and on freedom have been the topic of debate outside the immediate aim of developing feminist social theory (Taylor, 1986; Wapner, 1989). Although Foucault's work has been pulled into debates on relativism, his position is not an alignment with relativism but a thesis about the way that certain 'truths' can be the result and underpinning of power relations.[14] The perspective that is asserted in many of the critiques of Foucault is one that assumes that one has to seek the Truth, which will by definition be outside (or 'below', repressed by) power, in order to know what to do about changing present society. Hekman argues in defence of Foucault, that 'the assumption that political action, to be valid, must be founded in absolute values is precisely the assumption that Foucault is challenging' (1990: 180). Political action can never and need not be based on a fundamental and unchanging Truth. From a Foucauldian perspective, people enter into political action in the name of an historically specific truth, an unstable truth that their actions (both discursive and non-discursive) uphold. The values that political actions are based upon are for Foucault part of their discourse, not facts or Truths to be protected.[15] This is not the same as arguing that they are false and should henceforth be abandoned.

This 'unstable truth' would be the status of the universalised and naturalised category 'woman' in feminism. Foucault wanted to point out the way discourses create their own truths and the way that they are connected with the operations of power. Thus Foucault's point is not that all discourses that present their analysis in terms of the Truth, e.g. about how or where power operates in society, are wrong or false. His point is, first, that they are not straightforwardly outside of and against power because very often they are themselves based on power networks. Secondly, even if political actions produce the desired result, there may also be ramifications that could not be foreseen. With regard to developing alternatives to present power situations, he said:

> My point is not that everything is bad, but everything is dangerous, which is not exactly the same as bad. If everything is dangerous, then we always have something to do. So my position leads not to apathy but to a hyper and pessimistic activism. I think that the ethico-political choice we have to make every day is to determine which is the main danger.
>
> (1986a: 343)

Problems and frustrations arise because Foucault's analyses are much more present-orientated than the criticisms of his stance imply and demand. Foucault's strengths lie in his ability to pull apart the power and knowledge interconnections that have forged *present* truths, not in developing programmes of action for the future (which is not to say that he never spoke about action; he did: see Chapter 6). He is arguing not about any statement, but about those truths that *have* been generally accepted as true. As Hacking (1986) has argued, Foucault studied the empirical conditions under which truths are formulated, the 'totality of rules according to which the true is distinguished from the false and the concrete effects of power attached to what is true' (Foucault, 1981: 306). In order to interrogate present truths the critic does not *need* to appeal to a fundamental Truth that has been covered up, nor does s/he *need* a vision of what would improve on this truth (even if 'politically' s/he may have one).

Foucault's politics therefore has its emphasis on local resistance and the questioning of discursive categories that surround us. As Rajchman suggests, 'its motor is scepticism'; his philosophy is neither merely descriptive nor prescriptive but 'is occasion, spark, challenge. It is risk' (1985: 7, 123). There is no great Foucauldian plan for political critique, but there is the suggestion throughout his writings and interviews that one should be continually questioning the taken for granted truths that structure daily lives. This is a form of action in which Foucault suggested theorists should engage. This questioning includes questioning of one's own political discourse and the links with power that its knowledge base may entail.[16] He saw his work as that of the 'specific intellectual' who is 'attentive to the present', who 'locates and marks the weak points, the openings, the lines of force, who is incessantly on the move, who does not know exactly where he is heading nor what he will think tomorrow' (1988: 124).

Foucault argued that systems of constraint will always exist. It is in the ability to *change* them that he saw the possibility of political action (1988: 294). He does not posit a liberation that gets outside of power, but argues that power and freedom are not mutually exclusive. Power is analogous to a network, and the political problem is not to work towards some abstract freedom outside this network but to *negotiate* our lives, our freedom, within power. Rather belatedly, Foucault clarified his argument that power is not the opposite of freedom:

> Power is exercised only over free subjects, and only insofar as they are free. By this we mean individual or collective subjects who are faced with a field of possibilities in which several ways of behaving, several reactions and diverse comportments may be realised. . . . Consequently there is no face to face confrontation of power and freedom which is mutually exclusive.
>
> (1986b: 221)

In Foucault's eyes, therefore, his analyses of power and the power effects of discourse are already analyses of freedom. It

55

does not make sense to criticise him for failing to make space for freedom in his work.[17] For Foucault, power works 'within' freedom: freedom is not in the future or in the past but in the present.

Feminism is a movement of resistance *par excellence* in our society: often it entails movements Foucault would term 'reverse discourses'. Feminism can be understood as negotiating the freedom of women, making critiques of widely believed truths about women and making demands based on the feminist truths that presently seem correct and legitimate. Foucault's attack on claims to truth should not lead feminism into political paralysis: a Foucauldian feminism would be analysis that is determined in its critique at the same time as it acknowledges its ability to be proven wrong in its theoretical construction. As Hekman argues, it would be a feminist version of what Foucault calls a 'critical ontology of ourselves' (1990: 183). In order to avoid the same problems as the notion of 'experience', however, such an 'ontology' has to involve an historical interrogation of our construction, of what and how we 'know'. It is thus

> an attitude, an ethos, a philosophical life in which what we are is at one and the same time the historical analysis of the limits that are imposed upon us and an experiment in going beyond them.
> (Foucault, 1986a: 50, quoted in Hekman, 1990: 183)

3

FAMILIAR STORIES
The feminist analyses of incest

Sociologists and anthropologists have traditionally regarded incest as disruptive of the family and as therefore disruptive of social order. By contrast, feminism has suggested that, paradoxical as it may seem, incest is actually produced and maintained by social order: the order of a male-dominated society. Consequently, feminists have asked fundamentally different questions from previous writers and produced answers which relate to a different set of problematics. To a certain extent the problematics of incest are those of the body of feminist work on sexual violence as a whole: issues of power, the effects of abuse on women's perceptions of themselves, the construction of male sexuality, the popular representations of sexual crimes, and so on. So what is the relationship between this body of feminist work and the questions for feminism raised by Foucault discussed in the previous chapter? In this chapter I consider the feminist work on incest in relation to the more overtly theoretical issues between Foucault and feminism. I use the same three themes, power, sexuality and discourse. The purpose of the chapter is twofold. First I mean to suggest that the feminist analyses of incest are much more subtle than they have been given credit for. That is, by making explicit some of the implications of the feminist stance, feminist work on incest can hold its own in the face of what has been perceived by some as the threat of work such as Foucault's. Secondly, the purpose is to suggest that the work of Foucault does pose difficult questions and that these questions can prompt a healthy reevaluation of feminist arguments. Again, therefore, I am looking for analogous arguments as well as points of divergence.

POWER

Feminist analyses have approached the topic of incest as one of many abuses which can be grouped under the rubric 'violence against women'. Kelly (1988b) has proposed that these various abuses be understood as on a 'continuum' of male violence. Such a concept has enabled feminists to make connections between forms of abuse such as rape, domestic violence and sexual harassment. Less overt forms of abuse have also been placed on this continuum and been analysed as forms of violence against women. There is a threefold rationale behind extending 'violence' beyond the common sense use of the term to include these less overt forms such as exhibitionism (McNeill, 1987) or psychosurgery (Hudson, 1987). First, it places at the forefront of analysis women's experiences of these behaviours. However trivial exhibitionism may be depicted, for example, the women to whom it happens feel violated. The incidents constrain women's behaviour both at the time and in the future, and women limit their movements both geographically and temporally, in order to avoid the threat of sexual violence.[1] Secondly, all the various behaviours serve to convey the one message: 'you are merely women'. Thirdly, the extension of the term violence is made in order to draw attention to the sheer volume of male behaviours that constrain women's lives, i.e. that are oppressive to women. It is only when these instances are seen in their totality that an overall 'strategy' is revealed.

However, Liddle has argued that feminist work is in danger of over-using the label 'violence'; by collapsing the distinction between violence and 'oppressive behaviours' the feminist stance 'transforms "violence" into a residual category into which anything pernicious or degrading might be thrown' (1989: 766). Liddle is aware that there is an important political strategy in the use of the phrase 'violence against women'. Nevertheless, the criticism raises an important point about regarding incest as violence.

There can be no doubt that perpetrators of incestuous abuse physically injure and sometimes even kill the victims of their abuse.[2] Incest certainly is 'about' violence. However, feminist analyses of child sexual abuse, including incestuous abuse, report that 'most child sexual abuse is not violent' (La Fontaine, 1990), that 'force was rarely used as it was not necessary' (Herman with

Hirschman, 1981: 83). As Driver says, 'the practised incest offender usually aims to leave no marks' (1989: 182). The full-blown use of force is often not required because the abuser has other tactics at his disposal. *Threats* of violence toward the girl herself or another can form a part of these tactics (see Ward, 1984: 142, and La Fontaine, 1990: 78, where a father threatens to kill the girl's mother if she tells anyone what has been happening). Here I am in agreement with Liddle (1989: 766) in suggesting that threats of violence cannot be simply equated with violence: they are rather about command and authority. Other tactics used are: telling her that it is an education for later life, that it is normal, that he loves her, she is special, promising and giving gifts, using her confusion to make her feel like the one at fault (Herman with Hirschman, 1981: 85; Ward, 1984: 149).

Thus the feminist analyses do not in fact present incest as simply about violence: it is also about the operations of power. It is not necessary to distinguish between violent behaviour and oppressive behaviours as Liddle suggests; indeed, that critique seems to rely on exactly the common sense notion of violence that feminists are challenging. But whilst we can say that incest is on the continuum of violence, to give the impression that 'violence' is the only relevant conceptual term is misleading and damaging to the feminist case. It is helpful to maintain some conceptual distinction between violence and power. Such a distinction has a long sociological tradition. That tradition has distinguished between violence on the one hand and power on the other in order to illustrate that violence is often unnecessary; powerful groups or individuals do not need to resort to violence. At its most general the distinction is that power is much more subtle and discreet than violence. Foucault continues this perspective when he states 'power's success is proportional to its ability to hide its own mechanisms' (1981: 86). For Foucault power is 'actions upon actions'. That is, the one who is constrained (the abused in the example of incest) is maintained as an acting individual. The operation of power does not stop people acting (chains or locked cells are not always necessary), but acts instead upon their movements (Foucault, 1986b).

In this section I focus on the 'mechanisms of power' that feminist writers and women survivors have spoken about. I argue that the feminist analyses convey a picture of power that is *both* disciplinary and juridico-discursive, in Foucault's terms. The feminist analyses therefore retain both the newer and the 'archaic' models of power as described by Foucault. The retention of what Foucauldians would regard as the operations of juridico-discursive power is the most obvious point of conflict with respect to power, and this is where I shall begin my investigations.

Juridico-discursive power in feminist analyses of incestuous abuse

[H]e demanded respect. His word was law. Our mother could shout at us to get up, go to bed, eat, clear up, etc. and maybe take a swipe at us. But the worst she could do was to say 'I'll tell your father'. He had to be obeyed.

(An incest survivor, in Droisen, 1989: 73)

The argument of this section is that the feminist analyses depict the Father's[3] or the abusing relative's exercise of power in the way that Foucault describes the sovereign's exercise of power. It will be recalled from Chapter 2 that Foucault's concept of juridico-discursive power pictures power as a prohibitive force, laying down the sphere of the forbidden. I am not arguing that juridico-discursive power is at work in its prohibitive capacity; it is instead in the capacity to command and to receive obedience that abusers can be seen as exercising juridico-discursive power.

This mode of power is possible due to the position that the abuser so often has in relation to the child. His position gives him authority: children are expected to obey. This authority is not in any way unusual, but is the socially accepted authority that an adult and especially the Father has within a household. Some feminists have suggested that where incest occurs paternal dominance is often exaggerated. Herman and Hirschman argue that 'these fathers ... tend toward *abuses of authority* of every conceivable kind, and they not infrequently endeavour to secure their dominant position by socially isolating the family from the outside world' (1977: 41; emphasis added). Nelson reports that incest is most likely to occur where traditional roles are extreme and family members are seen as the man's property (1982: 6).

But the authority/obedience model of power is not confined to families in which incestuous abuse occurs. Feminist accounts stress that the households in which incest occurs do not differ greatly from other households. 'Normal' family structure is seen as contributing to the problem in feminist analysis of incest, in line with wider feminist critiques of the family (such as Barrett and McIntosh, 1982). Herman argues that the root of the incest problem is the male-headed household where 'the man expects to have his will obeyed as head of household, and expects his family to provide him with domestic and sexual services' (Herman and Hirschman, quoted in Nelson, 1982: 84). Moreover, that children, especially young children, are taught to display unquestioning obedience to adults, especially their parents, and to trust their parents more than other adults, serves to make child sexual abuse easier, to confuse the child and to deter her reporting the incident to anyone (Ward, 1984: 143, 149). The power of the Father is the power of 'seizure', which Foucault identifies with juridico-discursive power.

The sovereign exercised his right to life only by exercising his right to kill, or by refraining from killing. . . . Power in this instance was essentially a right of seizure: of things, time, bodies, and ultimately life itself.

(1981: 136)

Ward argues '[in] the incestuous family we find the most powerless of females, a girl-child, has become the sexual possession of the Father, the king in his castle lording it over his concubine' (1984: 193). Ward quotes researchers who have described the Fathers as 'tyrants, as exercising paternal dominance, as needing to appear the strong patriarch' (1984: 194). Butler too suggests that the aggressors saw their homes as their castles, just as Western culture informs them they are, where they are the unchallenged rulers (1985: 73). Within the family dominated by the Father, Daughters are 'young, dependent and constantly accessible' (Ward, 1984: 151). Echoing this argument, Dominelli states that incest is 'practised by individual men who wield tremendous authority over the individual girl' (1986: 9). Nelson quotes Rich Snowden, a leader of men's counselling groups in San Francisco, who states '[t]hese fathers acknowledge that they could do what they did only because they could make their children obey and could command silence' (1982: 88).

In this way, therefore, the feminist analyses of incest depict the power of the Father as in many ways similar to the power of the sovereign: a juridico-discursive power based on command and obedience. That Fathers have a certain amount of this accepted power in the Family means that their sexual abuse of children is not so much a deviation from normal familial relations as an illustration of them. Incest is an abusive way to exercise a familial power that is socially acceptable. This is what the feminist argument 'incest is the abuse of power/authority' conveys.

That the feminist accounts retain the juridico-discursive model should not lead us to dismiss them with reference to a Foucauldian standard. It would seem that, in terms of the survivors' accounts, this model of power is appropriate. The argument that notions of command and obedience are irrelevant here does not sit easily with these accounts. I would argue that a feminist analysis should retain these concepts in its theorising of power in incestuous abuse, not through any 'fear' of loosing feminism into a Foucauldian framework, but because they are *appropriate* to the analysis. (And as we shall see in Chapter 4, it is exactly in his discussion of incest that Foucault himself retains the model of juridico-discursive power in his own theorising, albeit in a different way from the feminist analyses.)

However, the feminist analyses also describe power's operations in ways that are more on a par with Foucault's concept of disciplinary power. The next section considers how the feminist analyses illustrate the operations of a 'disciplinary' power in the practice of incest, and suggests that there are therefore both modes of power in operation.

Disciplinary power in feminist analyses of incestuous abuse [4]

> The family-as-haven is an ideological construct that obscures the fact that for the Daughters (at least) the family is a prison.
>
> (Ward, 1984: 87)

> Is it surprising that prisons resemble factories, schools, barracks, hospitals, which all resemble prisons?
>
> (Foucault, 1979a: 228)

The family is not explicitly considered as a disciplinary institution in *Discipline and Punish*. However, Foucault muses parenthetically on the family's employment of disciplinary techniques:

'Discipline' may be identified neither with an institution nor with an apparatus; it is a type of power, a modality for its exercise, comprising a whole set of techniques, procedures, levels of application, targets. . . . And it may be taken over either by 'specialised' institutions . . . or by institutions that use it as an essential instrument for a particular end . . . or by pre-existing authorities that find it a means of reinforcing or reorganising their internal mechanisms of power (*one day we shall show how intra-familial relations, essentially in the parents–children cell, have become 'disciplined', absorbing since the classical age external schemata, first educational and then military, then medical, psychiatric, psychological*).

(1979a: 215–16; emphasis added)

The purpose of this section is not to propose any historically causal argument about the family's use or 'absorption' of disciplinary techniques. Nor is it being argued that the family is one of the enclosed disciplinary institutions, a 'discipline blockade' (1979a: 209). Rather, the argument is that the feminist analyses and women survivors' accounts describe experiences of incestuous abuse in ways which suggest that the abuse involved tactics of power reminiscent of Foucault's disciplinary power. Thus the power relations that 'imprison' the one who is being abused are not simply described as juridico-discursive power, the rule of the Father (the sovereign) over the powerless and therefore obedient child. The subtleties of power's operations that are present in the feminist analyses are analogous to those described by Foucault as disciplinary. I shall explore the feminist analyses in light of the three basic instruments of discipline: hierarchical surveillance, normalising judgement and the examination (Foucault, 1979a: 170–94).

Hierarchical surveillance

Discipline is a mode of power that works through observation. Those upon whom discipline is applied are rendered visible. The trap of visibility is described by Foucault through a discussion of the Panopticon (see Chapter 2). For the inmate in the Panopticon, power is both visible and unverifiable. It is visible due to the constant presence of the observation tower, yet it is unverifiable because s/he can never know when s/he is being observed. The inmate is totally seen without ever seeing, whereas the observer is able to see everything without ever being seen.

In the feminist accounts of incestuous abuse, surveillance recurs as a theme, or arguably as a mechanism, by which the bodies of the Daughters are caught within a power network. Sometimes this is literally the abusive Father watching without himself being in view, what Ward calls 'visual raping' (1984: 82). There are examples of fathers and brothers watching through holes in walls, of girls being watched dressing and undressing (Ward, 1984: 22, 55, 82). The spaces within the home that were once thought of by the Daughters as private (such as bathrooms or bedrooms) become spaces in which they can be watched so that they have to be constantly alert, just as the inmates of the Panopticon.

This is surveillance at its most obvious, in the form of voyeurism. Nor need the Father be hidden in order to have the disciplinary effect. The Daughter can still be viewed without being able either to reciprocate the gaze or to protest for reasons other than physical obstruction: for example, through fear of punishment, by not having the language or knowledge through which to articulate protest, or by not having the strength to reject this precarious and ambiguous attention from someone who may otherwise be an inattentive figure in their lives. On this last point, women have spoken of the continual forgiveness of and disappointment by their abusers (Armstrong, 1978), the precarious satisfaction that came from being special to someone when they were special to no one else (Herman and Hirschman, 1977: 747). Just as the observed in the Panopticon can never know the motivation behind the gaze, so the survivors speak of the tense unease the Father's (gaze) created. The 'seductive fathers' of whom Herman writes created great unease for their Daughters, who were unsure whether his attentions were motivated by affection or sexual intent (Herman with Hirschman, 1981: 109–25).

The power of the disciplinary technique of surveillance requires that the individual be aware that s/he is being watched, ensured in the Panopticon by the observation tower constantly before the inmate's eyes. This visibility of power should not be forgotten in emphasising the visibility of the observed. Kelly reports that despite the resistance of one incest survivor she spoke to, 'it did not stop her step-father masturbating in the sitting room in the knowledge that she would see him' (1988b: 173). Knowing that she could not avoid seeing him was a form of power exercised by the abuser. Thus the girl does not have to be the one observed in order to be the one abused.

Discipline works through the operations of a surveillance which is unverifiable. Because they can never be sure *when* they are the target of the gaze, the inmates behave *as if* they are always being watched. The unpredictability of further abuse recurs in survivors' accounts. This 'never knowing' placed the Daughters concerned in a constant state of anxiety. One woman says:

> [T]here was always a fear of it happening . . . the incidents become blurred because the fear of it happening became the overriding thing.
>
> (In Ward, 1984: 50)

Another asks:

> [C]an you imagine the terror of never knowing, when I would be sitting at the table doing my homework, coming home from school or getting ready for church, when my father would tap me on the shoulder and I'd turn around to find him grinning nervously, his face all red, standing behind me with an erection? . . . I still have nightmares that my father is going to touch me and I'll turn around and see him like that.
>
> (In Butler, 1985: 66–7)

The effect of his gaze, therefore, is to make the young woman watch over herself – Foucault's 'automatic functioning of power'. Even when the abuser is no longer alive, the gaze may still be felt:

> I felt as if he was behind me and I felt as though I was going to get banged in the neck for telling someone – and he'd been dead six years.
>
> (In Kelly, 1988b: 125)

Thus far the mechanism of surveillance can be seen to make the Daughters watch over themselves, to take precautions to avoid being caught by his gaze and the abuse that may follow. There is also another aspect of disciplinary power that is important in the feminist analyses. This is the fact of isolation for the sexually assaulted child. Like the individual within the Panopticon, she can see the tower before her, and is aware of his gaze falling upon her, but she is often unable to see 'sideways', to those who share a comparable position, either within the household or outside it. 'I thought I was the only one and they would think I was really weird' (in Droisen, 1989: 81). The realisation that one is not alone can be a source of further sadness and guilt. One woman says:

I thought I was protecting my younger sister from him. It wasn't until we were adults that I plucked up the courage to say to her, 'Did Dad do anything to you as well?' When she said 'Yes', I said, 'Oh God I thought I was protecting you.' I felt so guilty.

(In Droisen, 1989: 77)

For another it was a source of relief:

It wasn't until I was in my forties that I read an article about other women who had been through similar experiences. It was incredible to learn that I was not the only one. I was so relieved.

(In Droisen, 1989: 75)

Normalising judgement

Foucault argues that disciplinary power operates through 'normalising judgement' (1979a: 177–84). By this he means that punishment does not require a breach of a rule so much as a stepping outside 'acceptable behaviour' as judged by the institution. The contrast therefore is between, on the one hand, a rule in the form of 'thou shalt not' to which behaviour is referred and according to which one is either in line or in contradiction, and, on the other hand, a guideline presented as the ideal toward which one should strive. Thus the individual performances of children within a school will be compared against each other and against the projected performance to which it is deemed they should be conforming. The measurement of divergencies from the norm and between each other results in hierarchies, and punishments, although incorporating physical punishments of the judicial model, will be essentially corrective (1979a: 177–80). Conformity to the norm is desired and non-conformities are marked and punished with a view to correcting the deviation.

The effect of this mode of power is to impose an homogeneity since everyone is pushed toward the same behaviour, but at the same time it has an individualising effect because it measures individuals' divergencies from the norm. Normalising judgement, therefore, consists of 'perpetual penality . . . it traverses all points and supervises every instant in the disciplinary institutions, compares, differentiates, hierarchises, homogenises, excludes. In short, it normalises' (1979a: 183).

In some of the feminist analyses there is also a concept of normalisation where a subservient femininity is the norm. Rush argues that incestuous assault prepares the girl child for conventional femininity, a life of accepting subordination to the males around her.

> The sexual abuse of children is an early manifestation of male power and oppression of the female . . . [it is] an unspoken but prominent factor in the socialising and preparing of the female to accept a subordinate role . . . [it] prepares her to submit later to the sexual abuse heaped on her by her boyfriend, lover and husband.
>
> (1974: 71)

With the same sentiment, Jeffreys (1982) argues that child sexual abuse is a premature encounter with what girls will experience in adulthood. Responding to Kempe and Kempe's (1978) suggestion that incestuous assault may be overcome in girls but is ruinous for boys, Jeffreys argues 'the seriousness of childhood sexual experiences is assessed according to whether it reinforces or undermines the training of children into . . . power relations under male supremacy' (1982: 64). Herman also argues that in the group of women she spoke to, the daughters learnt not how to please themselves, but how to please a man: 'In short, they were well prepared for conventional femininity' (Herman with Hirschman, 1981: 118). Moreover, she suggests that 'incest represents a common pattern of traditional female socialisation carried to a pathological extreme' (1981: 125). The norm that is set up therefore is the subordinate, feminine, self-effacing woman.

Echoing this perspective, Ward argues:

> [M]ost Daughters are being prepared, overtly or covertly, for stereotypical femininity – which is based on dislike of women and aggrandisement of men. The patriarchal family

constructs Daughters who are ready, willing, and able to co-operate in male supremacist society. Father–Daughter rape is merely a phenomenon at one end of the spectrum by which this construction is achieved.

(1984: 196–7)

In other words, the way that abused girl children are treated by the abuser informs their understanding of themselves. Herman and Hirschman note that 'almost every one of fifteen women described herself as a "witch", "bitch" or "whore"' (1977: 751). Ward considers Lukianowicz's (1972) conclusion that some of the survivors 'became promiscuous' and argues that this should be understood as 'acting out the sexual object role that they had been given within the family' (1984: 154). Ward suggests that such a response should be seen as self-assertion. She argues that the survivors have been given status only as objects of sexual desire, and by being promiscuous or entering prostitution their behaviour flaunts the real status of women (1984: 155).

The survivor of incestuous abuse does not simply take on the label the Father's behaviour and words gave her, but his position in her life and his proximity make his influence predominate amongst the various ways which she could come to understand her self and her sexuality. One survivor reported 'he used to say "you want this" . . . that was drummed into me' (in Kelly, 1988b: 211). Another: 'that was when he started telling me I was a bitch and a slut and a cheap tramp. When I left home, that was what I thought I was, because I felt as though I'd let it all happen!' (in Ward, 1984: 70).

Thus the feminist analyses of incest see incestuous abuse as an extreme form of the training that all girl children receive. The normalising aim of such training is feminine, subordinate girls and women. Of course, a family may subvert such training, offering alternative femininities, challenging all or part of the norm of femininity. But in practice the family is frequently an important site for the training for or 'deployment' (De Lauretis, 1987) of femininity. This femininity may be considered similar to Foucault's concept of 'docile bodies', a pattern of behaviour that is docile not in the sense of being lazy, but to the extent that the body, whilst seemingly in control of its actions, acts in accordance with disciplinary power. The docile body is a useful body, forming part of the larger machinery. The 'larger machinery' may be 'normal' family structure, the construction of compulsory heterosexuality, or 'male supremacy'. The 'aim' of docile femininity is not consciously planned by the abuser. Nor is it bound to be 'successful' since those abused may resist the abuse and/or this deployment of gender. The feminist analyses of incest have shown how abused children often employ those tactics that are available to them to resist the abuse. She may run away, avoid being at home alone with him, feign sleep, tell someone (Kelly, 1988b; Gordon, 1988). She may make the connection with others and see her experience reflected in an empowering feminist discourse of sexual violence. But whilst girls and women may resist it, the 'deployment of gender' entails the lesson that the feminine body, as Bartky (1988) suggested, is not one's own. In incestuous abuse, this message is at its most literal.

The examination

[W]e were incest objects.

(Armstrong, 1978: 233)

In the examination, Foucault argues, the techniques of hierarchical observation and normalising judgement are combined. In the examination

> are combined the ceremony of power and the form of the experiment, the deployment of force and the establishment of truth. At the heart of the procedures of discipline, it manifests the subjection of those who are perceived as objects and the objectification of those who are subjected.
>
> (1979a: 184–5)

Incestuous abuse as an 'examination' in this sense might be a description of feminist analyses. Incestuous abuse is certainly a 'ceremony of power', on the different levels being discussed here. The disciplinary power of the Father's gaze but also his juridical power as sovereign are combined as the Daughter becomes the 'surface' of the Father's 'experiment'. It is she who is perceived as an object and whose objectification is revealed by her subjection to the abuse. The examination is the 'ceremony of this objectification' (1979a: 187).

The ceremony of disciplinary power had the form of the parade, the review, in which 'the subjects were presented as objects to the observation of a power that was manifested only by its gaze' (1979a: 188). It is the objectification so apparent in sexual abuse (in its many forms) that makes the notion of the objectification of female bodies so important to feminist analyses. But incestuous abuse can also be seen to have a productive effect or aim which is to produce a conventional femininity. The feminist position could be summarised thus: the subjectification process involved in incestuous abuse is one by which children are subjected to abuse and treated as objects such that they are subjectified as feminine[5] in the sense discussed above.

The notion of the abuser as sovereign returns in this discussion of discipline in the sense that incestuous abuse can be seen to combine both of the two forms of ceremony that Foucault associates with two different modes of power. In contrast to the disciplinary parade, the political ceremony of sovereign power was related to triumph:

> [I]t was a spectacular expression of potency, an 'expenditure', exaggerated and coded, in which power renewed its vigour. It was always more or less related to triumph. The solemn appearance of the sovereign brought with it something of the consecration, the coronation, the return from victory.
>
> (1979a: 187–8)

In incestuous abuse, the abuser appears as sovereign in the mode of judicial power and restates his position as the powerful one. The sexual abuse, moreover, may appear to the abused child as a triumph, that is, his triumph over her will. This is illustrated by Ward's argument that Father–Daughter incest is experienced as rape, and rape is 'the experience of powerlessness, of being conquered. The conquered territory is our own bodies' (1984: 118).

Summary

The incorporation of the tenets of disciplinary power into the analysis of power in incestuous abuse emphasises that in a feminist analysis abuse produces more than the immediate moment of subordination: it has effects beyond violence and the violation. Where there is violence, the Daughter's body may carry the mark of power in the most physical of senses. With the violation, the effects of incest can be extremely damaging in terms of psychological well-being. All of the feminist analyses agree on these two arguments. But the sociological argument that emerges from the feminist analyses is that the Daughter is *subjected to* and *subjectified through* the abuse in ways that continually attempt to place her within prevailing familial and gender relations.

Domination

One of the most important arguments of the feminist analyses is that incestuous abuse is a crime committed overwhelmingly by men against women. It is this 'perpetual asymmetry' that feminist analyses highlight and that may seem to drop out of the discussion as one, following Foucault, begins to concentrate upon how power is exercised as opposed to who is exercising it over whom.

As discussed in Chapter 2, Foucault does concede in a late interview that the 'strategic games' of power should be differentiated from 'states of domination' (in Bernauer and Rasmussen, 1988: 19).[6] It is clear that the notion of domination has a place in feminist analyses of incestuous abuse. The glaring asymmetry of the statistical evidence, such that it is, reveals a clear case of 'domination' of male over female and adult over child. Waldby *et al.* call this 'structural power':

> This form of power is hierarchical, static, public, socially legitimated (it has 'authority'); it is a form of control: the 'power over' model, with all its connotations of competition, dominance, and force.
>
> (1989: 102)

However, I suggested in the discussions of Foucault and feminism in the previous chapter that domination is best understood not as a backdrop 'behind' the operations of power but, rather, as built up through them. The distinction between these modes of conceptualising domination in respect to incestuous abuse is that in the first the abuse is understood within the context of that state of domination, in such a way that domination is not explained but theoretically presumed (Adams, 1979). It is rather the explanation of power relations, i.e. a focus on the tactics by which the perpetual asymmetry of power is upheld, that is being suggested here.

71

The two modes of power – the authority of the Father figure (juridico-discursive power) and the disciplinary tactics – make incestuous abuse possible and, together with the operations of power in other areas, build up the state of domination that exists between the groups male/female and adult/child (and especially parent/child). Thus although I would agree with Waldby *et al.* that there is a need to theorise what they term the structural level and I term domination, domination is not, as they characterise it, a static power, but is an asymmetry built upon the constant practice of power. Nor is it to be analytically collapsed into authority, for whilst authority and domination are linked in child sexual abuse, and especially in incestuous abuse, authority may not always be the sign of domination.[7]

SEXUALITY

In arguing that the offender is motivated by aggression, it is implied that he is not really interested in sexual gratification as such. The idea then develops that his behaviour is not *sexually* oriented at all. This allows us to avoid looking at any connections between male aggression and male sexual pleasure, and to avoid the uncomfortable thought that male sexuality in general may be implicated in the act.

(Driver, 1989: 13)

Where does sexuality fit into the feminist analyses of incest? The argument that incest is about power not sex was mainly a consequence of taking up the feminist model of rape as the paradigm for the analysis of incest. Early feminist analyses argued that rape was about power, both in terms of its motivation, where rape was theorised as a man wanting to assert power to feel dominant (Russell, 1975), and in terms of the power relations between men and women, which it simultaneously demonstrates and continues (Brownmiller, 1975). This 'not sex, power' position influenced feminist analyses of incestuous abuse. Herman, for example, argues that 'power and dominance rather than sexual pleasure may be the primary motivation [in incestuous abuse]' (Herman and Hirschman, 1981: 87). Waldby *et al.* argue that by 'linking the phenomenon of incest with the nature of the family and male–female relationships in patriarchal society' incest can be analysed according to a 'power theory' (1989: 101). However, there has been a certain muddying of the 'not sex, power' slogan in feminist theorising of rape, and the question of sexuality has been brought (back) into discussions of sexual assaults notably with the work of MacKinnon (I discuss these developments in more detail in Chapter 6). MacKinnon (1982; 1987; 1989) argues that one must situate rape within the context of heterosexual relations with particular attention to the 'normal' masculine role: '[the] male sexual role . . . centres on aggressive intrusion on those with less power. Such acts of dominance are experienced as sexually arousing, as sex itself' (1989: 127).

Similarly, a discussion of sexuality is crucial to analyses of incestuous abuse, as the quotation from Driver suggests, because of the ways in which sexual abuse implicates 'normal' masculine sexuality.

> These Fathers are not aberrant males: they are acting within the mainstream of masculine sexual behaviour which sees women as sexual commodities and believes men have a right to use/abuse these commodities how and whenever they can.
>
> (Ward, 1984: 194–5)

For feminists writing about incestuous abuse, the construction of normal masculine sexuality is a 'positive contributor to incest' (Nelson, 1982: 83). Whilst the feminist analyses of incest all share this general perspective, they do not spell out a theoretical position on the social construction of sexuality. Consequently the arguments tend to appear as mere assertions or as rather crude adoptions of a neo-Marxist position on ideology which portrays individuals as living out the ideological messages to which they are exposed.

Feminist work in other areas, however, has discussed the construction of sexuality more directly, and this work has been influenced by Foucault's arguments. In *THS*, sexuality is 'imbedded in bodies' by the operations of power/knowledge networks which have constructed it as a deep truth located within the individual. A later article clarifies Foucault's arguments on subjectivity, mostly implicit in *THS*. He argues that power operates to turn individuals into subjects:

This form of power applies itself to immediate everyday life which categorises the individual, marks him by his own individuality, attaches him to his own identity. . . . It is a form of power which makes individuals subjects. There are two meanings of the word subject: subject to someone else by control and dependence, and tied to his own identity by a conscience or self-knowledge. Both meanings suggest a form of power which subjugates and makes subject to.

(1986b: 212)

De Lauretis (1987) has used Foucault's framework to focus on the construction or deployment of gender as it occurs through processes of representation and self-representation. She argues that the construction of gender is 'both the product and the process of its representation and self-representation' (1987: 9). That is, the individual lives, or 'performs', in Butler's (1990a) term, the representation of gender as a self-representation, and that performance constitutes gender. The point here is that gender is informed by processes of representation or discourses. Discourses can refer to images seen as well as images heard. The individual who moves among these discourses, as well as adding to them, is constructed by them. De Lauretis draws upon the work of Althusser in her explanation of the process by which representation 'out there' becomes self-representation, part of a subject's performance of subjectivity. In particular she uses his notion of interpellation. Interpellation is the process by which individuals are 'hailed' by the discourse. That is, they 'recognise' themselves in the representation so that the representation can be said to inform or deploy their subjectivity.[8]

There are of course several different representations of masculine sexuality. The dominant representation, however, the one which is quintessentially male, is that of the predatory heterosexual man. Masculine sexuality is depicted as an aggressive force, easily tempted and, once roused, needing to be expressed. The feminist analyses of incest suggest that since such a representation is valorised in our culture we cannot be surprised that some men act out this representation as their self-representation. The argument is that men are taught to seek dominance through sexual contact (as in Russell's argument) and to find dominance sexually stimulating (as in MacKinnon's argument). In this way masculine sexuality is (in)formed through cultural representations of it, and abusive behaviour is not sharply distinguishable from accepted masculine behaviour.

The association of masculinity with domination, of sexual dominance with personal 'success' is all pervasive. . . . Generally boys and men learn to experience their sexuality as an overwhelming and uncontrollable force; they learn to focus their feelings on submissive objects, and they learn the assertion of their sexual desires and the expectation of having them serviced.

(MacLeod and Saraga, 1988: 41)

Although all men move amongst these discourses it would not be fair to say that these discourses on sexuality are the only relevant discourses which construct 'men'. Each man may be exposed to a variety of other discourses which produce him as a subject. As Henriques *et al.* stressed, subjects are dynamic because discourses are 'dynamic and multiple':

We use subjectivity to refer to individuality and self-awareness – the condition of being a subject – but understand in this usage that subjects are always dynamic and multiple, always positioned in relation to discourses and practices and produced by these – the condition of being subject.

(1984: 3)

Such a position allows for the variety in masculine sexuality, for as MacLeod and Saraga add:

[M]ale sexuality is not one-dimensional, and within a culture oppositional ideologies exist (for example, men as caretakers of their families, gentle lovers and protectors of their daughters), and have their impact on self-definition and cultural practices.

(1988: 41)

Thus although there are several ways in which masculine sexuality is informed, it is repeatedly represented in one particular way, a way which is valorised and which works to (in)form the self-representation of men in the realm of sexual behaviour, shaping their actions and their understanding of those actions.

De Lauretis stresses that the discourses that 'speak' to men contain a relational character. That is, representations of the masculine gender define masculinity in relation to femininity. When a man is 'hailed' by a representation he is placed within a category of people ('men') and in relation to another category of people ('women'). It is perhaps even more clear that representations of masculine heterosexuality are not just about 'male behaviour' but are also about the delineation of a relation between men and women. In predatory masculine hetero-sexuality this relation is at its most crude. Ward sums it up:

> Masculine sexual behaviour, as a social construct and, too often, as everyday practice, is devoid of tenderness, vulnerability and the fluid mutuality which flows from shared tenderness and vulnerability. *Masculine sexuality is inculcated in men and women alike as being concerned with conquering: 'getting a woman'.*
>
> (1984: 200; emphasis added)

The point here is that this representation of masculine sexuality entails a gender relation – 'getting a woman' – which is 'deployed' as part and parcel of the deployment of sexuality. This links up with Hollway's (1984) argument that discourses of sexuality are gendered. She argues that the various discourses which surround heterosexual relations work not just to construct the individual's understanding of his/her sexuality but also to position him/her in relation to members of the opposite gender. In the discourse of masculine heterosexuality under discussion here, women are objectified – 'getting a woman' – as men are simultaneously subjectified. In sexual abuse, the subjectification of the abuser and the objectification of the abused is immediate and graphic. Sexual abuse involves the level of male power Andrea Dworkin describes as an 'I am', what she terms a 'metaphysical assertion of self' (1981: 13). It has been argued that sexual murder can be analysed in terms of a project of 'masculine transcendence' (Cameron and Fraser, 1987). Cameron and Fraser point to the emphasis that has been placed in Western philosophy and literature on transcendence: 'the struggle to free oneself, by a conscious act of will, from the material constraints which normally determine human destiny' (1987: 168). This project informs masculine sexuality, where the 'motifs' are 'performance, penetration, conquest' (1987: 169). Sexual murder is the ultimate objectification, but in sexual abuse, too, the woman/child is treated as if she were an object.

As Ward suggests by her phrase 'in men and women alike', representations of sexuality are seen and heard by both men *and* women. Thus far I have concentrated on men's relationship to the discourses of masculine heterosexuality. However, women are also exposed to this representation of masculine sexuality in their daily lives. Women are not 'interpellated' by this construction in the way men are because they do not define it as 'speaking' to women. But this does not mean that women are not positioned in that discourse, nor that they ignore it. On the contrary, women are positioned as the objects of masculine sexuality and are therefore made to take account of it. For example, women watch over themselves, altering their geographical movements, as Hanmer and Saunders (1984) show, or dress according to this understanding of men's sexuality so as not to 'tempt' men. In this sense, the representation and self-representations of masculine sexuality as dominant, aggressive, spontaneous, etc. form a part of women's relationship to men as a group, just as it informs men's relation to women. Whilst it does not subjectify women in the same way as it does men it does 'deploy' a gender relation in which women are involved and to which women respond.

Whilst incest has been considered on the continuum of sexual violence the feminist analyses of incestuous abuse have also had a further relational aspect to explain. This is the age relation, and it has been analysed in much the same way as the gender relation, stemming from the observation that heterosexuality is repeatedly constructed in terms of a relationship between an older man and a younger woman. Rush documents media representations of the older man/younger girl combination. In film scripts

> from Mary Pickford and Shirley Temple to Tatum O'Neal, the little girl of the silver screen may have changed her costume, cut her curls ... but her relationship to men remained unaltered ... she still sacrificed for, pursued or reformed a father figure.... The little girl/grown man combination proved so successful that 'Daddy Long Legs', in which an orphaned child grows up and actually marries her rich, middle-aged benefactor, was adapted for film four times.
>
> (1980: 116–7)

In addition to this presentation of girl children as cute and

77

sexually provocative, Rush notes the representation of grown women as childlike, and the corresponding representation of strong women as unattractive (1980: 117). MacKinnon has argued that 'women's infantilisation evokes paedophilia' (1982: 530) and Driver argues that in several different arenas Western societies are 'paedophiliac': 'the child is made to look or act like a woman, and the woman made to look or act like a child' (1989: 23). This is 'such an everyday part of our lives that we hardly notice it – in a Shirley Temple or Marilyn Monroe film, or an adult woman's baby doll nightgown, for example, or the absurd coyness of those bikinis designed for toddlers' (1989: 23).

Driver quotes an abuser who said: 'Look at all the millions of dollars that are being spent by old bags trying to make themselves look young – why should I feel like a pervert for going for someone who is really young?' (1989: 13). In the feminist analysis, he is not a pervert, he is, as he himself recognises, representative of his culture. 'The offender is not out of the ordinary . . . he came from among us and is a mirror of our culture' (Sanford, quoted in Rush, 1980). In other words, he is perverse only to the extent that 'modern society is . . . in actual fact, and directly, perverse' (Foucault, 1981: 47). Chesler has noted the normality of the older man/younger woman pattern, suggesting that

women are encouraged to commit incest as a way of life . . . as opposed to marrying our fathers we marry men like our fathers . . . men who are older than us, have more money than us, more power than us, are taller than us . . . our fathers.
(Quoted in Herman with Hirschman, 1981: 57–8)

Where the abuse takes place within the household, the feminist analyses see an intersection of the discourse on male sexuality with discourses on children that represent them as possessions, in particular the possessions of their caretakers. An abuser's behaviour has to be related 'to the whole system of social values about sexuality and the family in which he exists' (Nelson, 1982: 75). Ward argues that girl children are especially regarded as the possessions of the father of a family (1984: 197). In father–daughter incestuous abuse, no other man's property is offended (Herman with Hirschman, 1981; Armstrong, 1987).

The feminist analyses, therefore, theorise incestuous abuse within the context of discourses which can be said to inform the abuse. Incest is theoretically placed at the intersection of discourses on predatory masculine (hetero)sexuality, children as sexually attractive and children as possessions. Feminists' work argues that the commission of incestuous abuse has to be understood with the 'normal' and 'acceptable' as its context.

DISCOURSE, KNOWLEDGE AND THE CONSTRUCTION OF PERSONAGES

It has been suggested that Foucault's concentration on the production of discourse is not applicable to women's situation, that silence is more relevant to women:

> Much of our feminist work . . . is beginning to show that silence is and has been to modern women's lives what Foucault has argued that knowledge and discourse are and have been to modern men's: the major product of the most significant power that shapes us.
>
> (West, 1989: 66)

Foucault did place silence within his thesis. He argues in *THS* that silence can form a part of discursive strategies:

> Silence . . . is less the absolute limit of discourse, the other side from which it is separated by a strict boundary, than an element that functions alongside things said, with them and in relation to them within overall strategies.
>
> (1981: 27)

West is justified in her criticism of Foucault to the extent that he does seem to neglect silence as he turns his attention to the ways in which sexuality has been 'put into discourse'. As West recognises, her argument is particularly pertinent to incestuous and child sexual abuse. Feminist writers have stressed both the silence that women survivors have had to keep (either due to threats, fears or because they are not heard when they do speak)[9] and the wider silence that has kept the nature of incestuous abuse secret. Rush (1980) refers to child sexual abuse as 'the best kept secret', the *Feminist Review* collective to 'family secrets' (1988) and Butler (1985) to a 'conspiracy of silence'.

Drawing attention to and breaking this silence has indeed been a part of the feminist task. However, feminists have not just pointed to a silence. One of the lines of feminist critique is that incest *has* been spoken about, but that it has been spoken about in mythologised ways. As Foucault's approach to sexuality would suggest, there has not been simply an imposition of silence around incest. It is not the case that no one has been talking about incest. The breaking down of the myths about incest has been a major part of the feminist work in this area. The myths are specific variants of those which surround all forms of violence against women (Kelly, 1988b: 34–6).

From myths to discourses

In this section I consider the feminist critique of the myths of incest, and argue that Foucault's work can provide pointers as to how these myths can be theorised. Such an analysis suggests that the myths are not simply falsehoods or operations of 'rape ideology' (Ward, 1984), but are a complex and contradictory overlapping of several different sorts of knowledges with different origins and different targets. The silence of women survivors, moreover, should be placed within the context of the ways in which incest *has* been spoken about and analysed in relation to them. As the 'speakouts' on incest have shown, several aspects of the disparate discourse on incest required the silence of the survivors in order to maintain credibility. It is on the basis of survivors' accounts that the feminist knowledge has been built, and that has created space for more survivors to speak out with the promise that they will be heard.

In *Incest: Fact and Myth* (1982), Nelson contrasts the feminist understanding of what incest is about with the myths of incest found in common sense understandings of incest and in medical/psychological theories and practices. This is also the style of critique in other feminist accounts of incest (e.g. Herman with Hirschman, 1981; Driver, 1989). The 'myths' of incest tend to be set up in opposition to the feminist accounts, as a block of non-feminist perspectives on incest. Ward (1984) covers many of the myths with her term 'rape ideology', and Dominelli (1989) with her term 'patriarchal ideology'. The feminist knowledge of incest is then used to illustrate the falsity of these myths. I want to do something different with the feminist criticisms. My investigation of this block of non-feminist arguments suggests that they have different targets, several 'origins' and manifesta-tions and may have different implications. As the discussions in

Chapter 2 have suggested, I resituate the feminist critique within a perspective which does not regard these ways of talking about incest as simply myths, but seeks to map out the ways in which they function in relation to each other and according to larger strategies. Labelling all non-feminist discourses as myths misses the opportunity to explore their varied relations with respected knowledges and institutions.

One important division to make within these 'myths' is between those ways of talking about incest which construct the object 'incest' as something other than would a feminist knowledge, and those which, although in important ways converging with the feminist knowledge in what they see, diverge from a feminist knowledge in what they see incest as 'about'. The first way of speaking about incest denies its occurrence, denies it as a problem and/or locates incest geographically as a cultural practice. Nelson notes the many different areas in which she was assured incest was a 'way of life'. These ways of speaking are on a par with Foucault's 'old' ways of speaking about sex, in the sense that they seek not to surround and generate knowledge about incest, but to deny it as a problem.

The second type of 'myth' is in a sense the more pernicious because it acknowledges that incestuous abuse occurs, and more or less accepts that the form it takes amounts to child sexual abuse. Yet these myths construct incest as 'about' phenomena other than those that feminists place at the centre of attention. They are ways of talking which, although they may have disparate origins, frequently problematise incest in such a way that it is drawn into a medico-psychological domain. The structure of the following discussion is similar to that adopted by several of the feminist writers in that it is divided according to the separate targets that are constructed through the various ways of talking about incest.[10] Again, this exercise places a framework around what feminist accounts have already argued, an exercise that uses Foucault's notion of the strategies of the deployment of sexuality in a rewriting of feminist accounts. It will be recalled that Foucault's four strategies were: the psychiatrisation of perverse pleasures; a hysterisation of women's bodies, a pedagogisation of children's sex and a socialisation of procreative behaviour (1981: 104–5).

The perverse male

The feminist analyses have been critical of the notion that the person who abuses children is deviant, or, more specifically, a sexual 'pervert'. It will be clear from the above discussions that the feminist analyses have argued that the incest abuser is not sexually perverted, but is acting within the parameters of normal masculine sexuality. Feminists have argued that the depiction of the abuser as a pervert is a myth repeated in common knowledge as well as in academic explanation and treatment programmes. Ward quotes Weinberg, a sociologist, who states that

> [incest] is a behaviour that disrupts or destroys the social intimacy and sexual distance upon which family unity depends. It is the recourse of very disturbed and *very perverse* persons.
>
> (1951, quoted in Ward, 1984: 92; italics added)

Nelson quotes a study which depicted the man as deviant: it reported that half the sample of incest offenders were alcoholics 'and a great many more were imbeciles' (1982: 76). Some writers have even found 'atrophy of the frontal lobe' (1982: 76). Nelson lists the sexual perversities these men have been said to have: they are 'undersexed, oversexed, unconscious homosexuals, uninhibited heterosexuals' (1982: 76). One recent study which clearly sets up its questions in a way that defines the problem of incest as a sexual response is entitled 'Erectile Responses among Heterosexual Child Molesters, Father–Daughter Incest Offenders, and Matched Non-Offenders: Five Distinct Age Preference Profiles' (Barbaree and Marshall, 1989).

Trying to identify a particular sexual preference in incest offenders drastically misses the ways in which normal sexuality, normal power relations and the normal family are implicated in incestuous abuse. The men who are known to have abused children are not perverted, but 'normal', everyday men:

> The aggressors are not outcasts and strangers; they are neighbours, family friends, uncles, cousins, stepfathers and fathers.
>
> (Herman with Hirschman, 1981: 7)

In the case histories that I have read, and from women I have talked to, it is obvious that the Fathers come from every class in society. A judge, a barrister, a diplomat, an eminent doctor, a university lecturer, a teacher, a university student, a business man, a film star, a labourer, a tradesman, a public servant, a farmer, a counsellor, a minister of religion, a soldier, a politician, unemployed, handicapped, very old, very young: Every man.

(Ward, 1984: 87)

The point is not that perverted men are in every walk of life but that the distinction normal/perverse describes a qualitative distinction in sexuality. In effect the feminist analyses accuse those who regard the incest offender as perverted of making the move from act to species that Foucault outlined in relation to the deployment of sexuality. By creating a distinction between the normal male and the incest offender that appeals to a notion of perverted sexual desire, this discourse perpetuates a way of speaking about incest that fails to acknowledge or investigate the ways in which both the normal and the abnormal are produced by similar, even the same, 'acceptable' discourses.

The colluding mother

Foucault argues that the 'hysterisation' of women's bodies included the assertion that the feminine body 'produced and had to guarantee [the life of children], by virtue of a biologico-moral responsibility lasting through the entire period of the children's education' (1981: 104). Feminists have highlighted the ways in which the mother of an incestuously abused child is repeatedly depicted as incompetent. Not only are her mothering abilities judged, but her 'incompetence' has led her to be held in some part responsible for the abuse.

[A husband may be given] an extra push by a wife who arranges situations that allow privacy between father and daughter. She may, for example, arrange her work schedule so that it takes her away from home in the evenings, and tell her daughter to 'take care of dad'.

Stories from the mother that they could not be more surprised can generally be discounted – we have simply not seen an innocent mother in long-standing incest, although the mother escapes the punishment that her husband is likely to suffer.

(Both from Kempe and Kempe, quoted in Nelson, 1982: 55, 56)

Nelson notes that when the mothers are not depicted as collusive, they are depicted as spiteful: '[When] wives report the incestuous liaison it is not so much because they object to the incestuous act, but because they are angry over some other matter' (Henderson, quoted in Nelson, 1982: 56). In these mother-blaming arguments, the mother is drawn into the psychiatrisation of families in which incest occurs. She is cast as an inadequate mother in parallel with the man's depiction as a sexual pervert. Armstrong notes this trend to build 'the "profile" of the "incest mother"' (1987: 265). Her sexual service to the man is often central in these descriptions:

> She keeps herself tired and worn out. . . . She is frigid and wants no sex with her husband. This is another way of bowing out of her role as a wife, and giving reason to the husband to look elsewhere for sex.
>
> (Justice and Justice, quoted in
> Herman with Hirschman, 1981: 43)

Herman notes further comments of 'experts' on mothers in households where incestuous and child abuse have occurred. Cromier, a psychiatrist, described the mothers as 'frigid, hostile, unloving women'; Walters, an 'expert on child abuse', described them as 'very unattractive' (both quoted in Herman with Hirschman, 1981: 43).

These constructions form part of a larger strategy that punishes women for not fulfilling the role of the all-seeing Mother whose biological-moral responsibility is to protect her children, suggesting that she was either negligent or incapable of this 'duty'. Explanations of her behaviour make an implicit appeal to this mothering role from which she has erred, and as a consequence she is presented as not a 'real' woman/Mother. The feminist position is not that mothers are never irresponsible, but that the the image of the 'responsible mother' against which women are judged is one that serves to cast them as unfeminine, even unnatural (how *could* she?). By suggesting that these women are of a particular type, psycho-medical discourse attempts to create a discursive divide much like the responsible Mother/nervous woman that Foucault sketched out, a division which continues a longstanding way of speaking about women.

The seductive daughter

Foucault suggests that a further strategy of the deployment of sexuality was focused on the dangers of children's sexuality: 'Parents, families, doctors and eventually psychologists would have to take charge, in a continuous way, of this precious and perilous, dangerous and endangered sexual potential' (1981: 104). The feminist analyses of incest trace the various ways in which the abused child is held responsible for the abuse. One predominant way that the girl child is spoken about is as seductive and sexually forward. Ward argues that there is widespread belief in the 'Lolita syndrome' (1984: 139), named after the girl in Nabokov's novel who 'seduces' an adult man. One oft-quoted paper argued:

> These children undoubtedly do not deserve completely the cloak of innocence with which they have been endowed by moralists, social reformers and legislators . . . these children were distinguished as unusually charming and attractive . . . frequently we considered the possibility that the child might have been the actual seducer, rather than the one innocently seduced.
>
> (Bender and Blau, 1937, quoted in Ward, 1984: 90)

A crude interpretation of Freud's work has encouraged this depiction of the child as responsible for tempting the abuser. It is now well known that Freud initially suggested that childhood sexual trauma had a role to play in the development of 'hysteria' in adult women (Freud and Breuer, 1956). Later, however, he retracted this theory, substituting instead the argument that his patients were verbalising their incestuous *fantasies* (Masson, 1985; Arens, 1986). Freud argued that all children unconsciously desire their opposite sexed parent, and that the psychic 'resolution' of this Oedipal complex, imperfect as this resolution may be, is a normal part of development.

Much clinical work that has dealt with cases of actual incestuous abuse has been carried out in the shadow of such a theory, regarding the daughter as acting out incestuous desires which would normally be at this point repressed during a period of latency. One research team saw the sexual fantasies and ambiguity of Oedipal desires of the girl child as realised in the imprisonment of the abuser: 'Since the sexuality of these girls led to the arrest and incarceration of the father and disruption of the home, they had the experience of seeing their destructive, omnipotent fantasies come true' (Kaufman *et al.*, 1954, quoted in Ward, 1984: 148). More recently, in 1975, it has been argued:

> Although pubic and professional sentiment is generally empathetic toward the daughter and negative toward the father, there are indications that the daughter may play an active and initiating role in the incestuous relationship . . . the daughter is usually the *passive* participant who seldom complains or resists.
>
> (Sarles, quoted in Ward, 1984: 157; her emphasis)

In this way the girl child is depicted as cooperating in the abuse. Nelson quotes Leroy Schultz, who has argued that '[b]oth offender and victim are symbiotic or form a cooperative dyad' (1982: 40), and Ward quotes Weiner, who in 1962 wrote: there is much to show 'that the daughters, like their mothers, are not merely innocent pawns of their father's will' (1984: 148). Ward notes a contradiction much like Foucault's 'double assertion'; children are non-sexual until there is an accusation of incestuous abuse, at which they become sexually provocative.

> It is a curious fact that it is generally conservative thinking which regards children as innocent non-sexual vessels who must be coddled and protected . . . and yet it is the same conservative view which treats the Daughter as She-Devils in the guise of children – especially when the public reputation of the father is threatened.
>
> (1984: 148)

The sexuality of children is a subject which sits uneasily in current Western discourses on sexuality. The subject attracts these contradictory statements presenting children as simultaneously sexual and not sexual, as innocent and as provocative. The feminist arguments around incestuous abuse highlight the ways in which children are understood only in reference to a wicked/innocent mould. Kitzinger (1988) has warned feminists against using that same distinction in arguments against child sexual abuse; we cannot simply assert that children are 'innocent victims' because this risks continuing an understanding of children that can work against a 'knowing' child. Rather, the idealisation of a certain representation of childhood needs to be challenged, and the subject of incestuous abuse needs to depart from the constructions participant/victim and provocative/innocent.

Implications

This exploration highlights the fact that the non-feminist discourse on incest draws on knowledges with very different origins including different schools of psychology, literature and 'common knowledge'. The different psychological theories span psychoanalytic, systemic family therapy and behavioural explanations. They converge and are implicated in the emergence of the various personages discussed above. In the same way that the operations of the deployment of sexuality described by Foucault create and deploy different personages, so these ways of speaking about incest construct the 'perverted father', the 'colluding mother' and the 'seductive daughter'. Once these figures are constructed the move to the 'dysfunctional family' is not very far. Originating from systems theory, this perspective regards the family as a whole as dysfunctional, each member contributing through repeated behaviours to the continued dysfunction. Such a theory has been widely criticised by feminists, especially with regard to its normalising effects. That is, the dysfunctional family theory implies that there is a healthy family system. It has, moreover, a narrow focus on family members' interactions, a non-blaming approach which gives responsibility to the family's interactions as a system not to an individual member of the family, and a consequent lack of direct challenge to the family as an institution in which power is unequally exercised. Within family therapy theory, it has been argued, the social construction of power and gender within the family are ironically treated like 'family secrets' (Hare-Mustin, 1987: 25).[11]

Just as Foucault suggested that the Malthusian couple – the fourth strategy of the deployment of sexuality – has been deployed and normalised, so the feminist analyses suggest that a familial system entailing gender differentiated roles and responsibilities has been upheld within discourses around incestuous abuse. The difference between them, of course, is that Foucault's position implies that 'the family' is not deployed as a whole but is constituted through the several discourses. The feminist position, on the other hand, tends to speak of the normalisation of 'the family' as a hegemonic ideology, a totalised way of speaking that obscures the oppressive realities of family life.

The non-feminist discourse on incest is a complex web of interlocking knowledges and ways of talking about incest. To discount these with the blanket term 'myths' or 'male ideology' is to ignore the ways in which these various ways of talking interrelate and conflict, and the institutional and power relations they deploy and inform. To ignore this complexity misses the opportunity to expose these interconnections, to investigate historical tactics and mechanisms, and to use the points of conflict to question the wider issue of making truth claims about incest. These ways of speaking about incest are tied, moreover, to concrete practices. Most explicitly in clinical settings the knowledge of incest that arises is based on the work of practitioners and is implemented in their work. The knowledges of incest often inform practices which involve the exercise of power; they are 'made to function as true'. Thus it is not simply that these ways of talking about incest are myths, that they are wrong, but that they constitute knowledges, often institution- alised as truths with practices informed by and informing them. It is arguably their base in respected knowledges and institutional settings that makes these ways of speaking so tenacious: it is here that explorations need to focus.

Feminist knowledge and subjugated knowledges

An important question for this rewriting is where to place the feminist knowledge of incest and the survivors' discourse which forms a solid basis for the feminist analyses. In Chapter 2 I discussed the possible antithesis between Foucault and feminism on claims to truth. It is clear that in the work on myths the feminist analyses of incest are involved in the 'deconstruction of truths' as advocated by Smart (1989). However, the feminist analyses might be seen to be setting up another Truth of incest in contrast to the falsity of the various myths; such an approach is explicit in the 'fact and myth' of Nelson's title. Through the critique of the 'myths' of incest the feminist work simultaneously constructs its version of what incest is really 'about'. But such a claim to authority is problematic within the Foucauldian framework. The issue is the status of the feminist analyses of incest. In the remainder of this section I want to argue not that feminism can get around this problem, but that the reflexivity to which it leads forces feminists to ask: How do feminists decide what incest is 'about'?

Feminist analyses of incest are based in large part on the survivors' accounts that have been given over the past fifteen years or so. These accounts can be regarded as 'subjugated knowledges' in Foucault's sense. Foucault spoke of subjugated knowledges as 'disguised' in a way which recalls the lack of acknowledgement of incestuous abuse in the theorisings of sociologists, psychologists and anthropologists: '[Subjugated knowledges are] those blocks of historical knowledge which were present but disguised within the body of functionalist and systematising theory and which criticism . . . has been able to reveal' (1980a: 82).

The survivors' accounts have been either ignored or reinterpreted in the discourses of psychology or medicine. Feminism, instead, takes them as its starting point, the foundation for its critique of other ways in which incest has been understood. The survivors' accounts are 'subjugated knowledges' to the extent that they fit Foucault's description:

[K]nowledges that have been disqualified as inadequate to their task or insufficiently elaborated: naive knowledges, located down on the hierarchy, beneath the required level of cognition or scientificity. I also believe it is through the reemergence of these low ranking knowledges, these unqualified, even directly disqualified knowledges (such as that of the psychiatric patient, the ill person, of the nurse, the doctor – parallel and marginal as they are to the knowledge of medicine – that of the delinquent, etc.) and which involve what I would call popular knowledge though it is far from common sense knowledge, but is on the contrary a particular, local, regional knowledge, a differential knowledge incapable of unanimity and which owes its force only to the harshness with which it is opposed by everything surrounding it – that it is through the reappearance of this knowledge, of these popular knowledges, these disqualified knowledges, that criticism performs its work.

(1980a: 82)

The survivors' accounts have been directly disqualified, most explicitly as fantasies by adherents to the Freudian legacy, and are indeed opposed to other ways of talking about incest. Their reemergence has formed, moreover, the basis of the feminist critique of ways of talking about incest. Using the survivors' accounts gives feminism a strong foundation for such a critique. However, it is the move from critique to theory that is problematic. The worry is whether feminist knowledge can escape becoming a self-appointed authority reminiscent of those myths and 'knowledges' to which it was originally opposed (Gunew, 1990).

However, the feminist analyses of incestuous abuse do not seek to set themselves up as the guardians of the access to Truth and objectivity. Although feminist analyses are empirical in the sense that they are based in the main upon women's oral evidence, they are not empiricist in the sense that they regard the social world as simply there to be accurately described. As discussed in Chapter 2, an embrace of Foucault's claim that knowledge is tied to power relations and can deploy power relations as it is used does not mean that feminism is unable to make claims to truth, but that feminism has to admit and be aware of its connections with power. The feminist work on incest is already reflexive about its claims to knowledge, and the politics of its language. The substitution of the term 'survivor' for 'victim' to convey the strength that these women have displayed as well as the various renamings of incest are examples of the reflexivity that feminism has displayed in this area.

Feminism has been sensitive to the unintended implications of its language. The feminist analyses of incest are necessarily reinterpretations of the 'subjugated knowledges' of survivors.[12] As such, they are not objective truths but feminist truths, built on the foundation of survivors' accounts, but not identical with them.[13] The feminist truths can be and are altered as more information comes to light. This knowledge is the one on which feminists base their critique and their actions. Such a stance is not one which accepts all ways of speaking as equally valid, that 'accepts the dominant group's insistence that their right to hold distorted views . . . is intellectually legitimate' (Harding, 1987: 295). It is in the first instance a descriptive stance. It notes that others do hold opposing views, ones that feminists would regard as mistaken or irrelevant, but is also aware of its own process of knowledge formation, avoiding setting itself up as an immutable Truth. Feminist knowledge of incest has a firm foundation in the survivors' accounts, but this does not mean that it is fixed and unable to adapt to new information.

4

TELLING AND TABOO
Feminism within the Foucauldian landscape

> [I]n a society such as ours, where the family is the most active site of sexuality, and where it is doubtless the exigencies of the latter which maintain and prolong its existence, incest . . . occupies a central place.
>
> (Foucault, 1981: 109)

In a few pages of *THS* Foucault sketches a bold argument on the subject of incest. Indeed, he situates incest in a pivotal position in the thesis of the book. His argument does not relate to who commits incest, its extent or location, but, as one would expect, is about the ways in which incest is put into discourse. Making his familiar manoeuvre, Foucault reflects upon the varied discourse on incest and how it corresponds to other ways of talking about sex; in doing so, he provides a template for a discussion that pulls together various constructions of incest. That is, his arguments can act as a place to gather and compare the sociological, anthropological, legal, welfarist and feminist discourses on incest.[1] This chapter discusses Foucault's comments on incest, and uses these arguments to pose two questions for feminist work on the subject. These questions concern the place of this feminist work within the landscape Foucault describes. First I ask: is the feminist work part of the deployment of sexuality? That is, does the talk it generates inscribe its participants into the power/knowledge networks Foucault details in *THS*? Secondly: what is the relationship of the feminist work to what went 'before' the deployment of sexuality, i.e. the deployment of alliance, which had its emphasis on kinship and prohibitions? Or, to focus this second question differently and more specifically: what has happened to the notion of the incest taboo in feminist work on incest?

THE INDISPENSABLE PIVOT: FOUCAULT ON INCEST

In Foucault's thesis incest is situated at a discursive crossroads between the deployment of sexuality and the deployment of alliance that preceded it. What does this mean? It will be recalled that there are two sorts of powers that have been exercised over sex, according to Foucault: first, the juridico-discursive mode, a prohibitive power that divides forbidden sexual acts from the permitted; and second, the proliferating and productive power of power/knowledge strategies and networks. These two powers correspond, furthermore, to two different ways by which people, as sexed bodies, have been related to each other: the deployment of alliance and the deployment of sexuality respectively. Most work on Foucault has concentrated upon the deployment of sexuality and the bio-politics associated with it. When considering the place of incest in Foucault's work, however, it is crucial to also bring the deployment of alliance into the picture (and with it comes an acknowledgement of continuing operations of juridico-discursive power) because what is special about incest in Foucault's thesis is that it traverses both deployments.

The deployment of alliance related people to each other through kinship. People were positioned with respect to others through a system of 'marriage, of fixation and development of kinship ties, of transmission of names and possessions' (1981: 106). This system revolved around human reproduction and blood ties; the concern was who was related to whom. The aim of the deployment of alliance was the reproduction of the institution of marriage and kinship systems. Within this network, the constraints placed on sexual behaviours or arrangements were on those which threatened the continuation of the system, such as adultery, bigamy and, of course, incest. The quality of family life is not a factor in the deployment of alliance: it is concerned only with the maintenance of lines of descent and systems of marriage. Thus it had an homoeostatic aim and function, always working to reproduce the social body in the same form.

Since the eighteenth century, however, Foucault suggests that the deployment of sexuality has been superimposed on the deployment of alliance. The deployment of sexuality is also a network linking people as sexual beings, but it relies upon different mechanisms of power and has different effects. The reproduction of past structures is no longer a goal of the network. Nor does the deployment of sexuality use mechanisms of constraint, repressing those behaviours that threaten the stability of the system. Instead, the deployment of sexuality works to expand and proliferate, operating through mobile and polymorphous techniques of power, monitoring sexualities not to punish but to measure pleasure:

> The deployment of alliance has as one of its chief objectives to reproduce the interplay of relations and maintain the law that governs them; the deployment of sexuality, on the other hand, engenders a continual extension of areas and forms of control. For the first what is pertinent is the link between partners and the definite statutes; the second is concerned with sensations of the body, the quality of pleasures.

> (1981: 106)

Although Foucault argues that the deployment of alliance has not been completely supplanted, that it is still at work and still important, it is clear that he believes it has been sufficiently eclipsed by the deployment of sexuality for the latter to now be considered the predominant mode of power's operations over sex. The process of change from one to the other centres on the family, the place where both 'systems' converge. Just as Marx argued that the relations of production of a new society matured within the framework of the old, so Foucault argues that the deployment of sexuality was constructed around and on the basis of the deployment of alliance (1981: 107).

The family, Foucault proposes, was the privileged institution of the deployment of alliance; it was the family structure that the system of alliance sought to maintain. It was also, he contends, the cornerstone in the establishment of the deployment of sexuality. Around the family there converged a variety of knowledges concerning sexual behaviour. These 'intrusions' into the family worked to map out the discrete sexualities contained within that unit. For example, the production of 'childhood sexuality' was set in motion, in part, by the exhortation to parents to beware the dangers of children's masturbation, which consequently drew a line between the sexuality of adults and children within the family unit. In this way many of the strategies of the deployment of sexuality worked through and were supported by the family, so that the family behaved as 'a crystal', seemingly the source of sexuality, but actually only reflecting and refracting the operations of the deployment of sexuality all around it (1981: 111). Thus the family was pivotal in the operations of the deployment of sexuality as a vehicle and site of its operations: its role was and is to 'anchor sexuality and provide it with permanent support' (1981: 108). By disseminating and sustaining the strategies surrounding sexuality, the family was 'one of the most valuable tactical components of the deployment [of sexuality]' (1981: 111). In sharp contrast with traditional histories of the Victorian era which see the family's role as one of constraining and excluding sexuality, Foucault argues that the family supports and intensifies the deployment of sexuality: sexuality is 'incestuous from the start', tied as it is to the institution of the family.

For Foucault, therefore, the family and incest are connected in two contrasting ways. In the deployment of alliance, incest is tied to the family because it is a sexual activity which needs to be prohibited for the family structure and the alliance system as a whole to continue. In the deployment of sexuality, incest is tied to the family because the family is the site at which many of the strategies which deploy sexuality first operate. In this sense, therefore, incest is placed at the crossroads between the two deployments.

Foucault is not merely arguing that incest 'belongs' to both deployments. He argues that incest is an irresolvable point of tension between the two systems. The tension arises, he contends, because whereas the deployment of alliance forbids incest, the deployment of sexuality actually incites it. There are two senses in which the discourses of the deployment of sexuality might incite incest. First, Foucault might mean that all the talk around the family as a place where sexuality develops and expresses itself incites further talk, including talk about incest, i.e. as a social problem, a potential social danger. Feminist discourse on incest would be one of the discourses to which Foucault's argument refers. From this perspective, feminist concern about the dangers of sexual abuse in the family becomes less a radical challenge to the family institution than merely another 'social problem' discourse alongside several other ways of talking about the family and sexual dangers.

Yet Foucault also seems to be making the stronger argument

that the practice of incest is actually incited by the operations of the deployment of sexuality. He suggests that because the strategies of the deployment of sexuality operate at their greatest intensity around the family, incest looks set to become the least remarkable of sexual practices. Taking the example of children's sexuality, he explains, in a later interview, how the discourses of the deployment of sexuality work to sexualise the family, and thereby to incite incest. He refers to parenting manuals that were produced in the eighteenth century instructing parents on the dangers of childhood sexual activity:

> One might argue that the purpose of these discourses was precisely to prevent children from having a sexuality. But their *effect* was to din it into parents' heads that their children's sex constituted a fundamental problem in terms of their parental educational responsibilities, and to din it into children's heads that their relationship with their own body and their own sex was to be a fundamental problem as far as they were concerned; and this had the consequence of sexually exciting the bodies of children while at the same time fixing the parental gaze and vigilance on the perils of infantile sexuality. The result was the sexualising of the infantile body, a sexualising of the relationship between parent and child, a sexualising of the familial domain.
>
> (1980a: 120)

When Foucault suggested that the deployment of sexuality incites incest, therefore, it seems he did not merely mean that a 'discursive space' was opened up for *talk* about the practice of incest, but that the discourses on sexuality that converged around the family incited the actual *practice* of incest. Thus the deployment of sexuality creates a problem for itself; although it 'needs' the family as the anchor for its discourses, it also threatens the family through its operations by inciting incest. Foucault suggests that the deployment of sexuality requires that an incest prohibition still operate and this is the point at which the deployment of alliance becomes important again.

> [I]ncest . . . is being constantly solicited and refused; it is an object of obsession and attraction, a dreadful secret and an indispensable pivot. It is manifested as a thing that is strictly forbidden in the family insofar as the latter functions as a

deployment of alliance; but it is also a thing that is continuously demanded in order for the family to be a hotbed of constant sexual incitement.

(1981: 109)

The incest prohibition is a straightforward example of juridico-discursive power: it is prohibitive and it is clearly discursive, a negative instruction 'thou shalt not'. It is, Foucault suggests, fundamental to the deployment of alliance, maintaining family roles and the rule of exogamy. From within the deployment of sexuality, therefore, there is a conservative force which still reiterates rules and prohibitions that are more akin to the deployment of alliance. This continuation of a way of talking that is becoming increasingly archaic is not merely a response to the incitement of the deployment of sexuality but is required by it. The deployment of sexuality requires the family, and it therefore also requires the incest prohibition.

This is the context in which Foucault understands the West's 'obsession' with the universality of an incest taboo. This may be, he argues, a defence against the deployment of sexuality which overwhelms the rules of the system of alliance. Feeling the effects of the deployment of sexuality, the 'affective intensification of family space' (1981: 109), as the knowledges and experts crowd around the family watching out for signs of sexuality and making the family watch itself, may have led, Foucault suggests, to this insistence that this one rule, the incest prohibition, was the universal rule of all rules. In this way the system of alliance 'resists' the deployment of sexuality and the deployment of sexuality clings onto the deployment of alliance. Although in the past two centuries Western societies have created many technologies that are foreign to the concept of law, Foucault suggests the proliferation of the newer forms of power are feared and, in the case of incest, the comparative safety of legal formulations (such as 'thou shalt not commit incest') is sought once again; thus there is an 'endless reworking of the trans-cultural theory of the incest taboo' (1981: 109–10). This results in a continual and unique tension around the issue of incest. It is an issue that sustains both deployments within one temporality. The incest prohibition is a part of the deployment of alliance that lingers on within societies in which the deployment of sexuality now predominates.

In a later interview Foucault takes his argument further and argues that the universal incest prohibition is a *recent* creation of certain discourses:

> Incest was a popular practice, and I mean by this, widely practised among the populace, for a very long time. It was towards the end of the 19th century that various social pressures were directed against it. And it is clear that the great interdiction against incest is an invention of the intellectuals. . . . If you look for studies by sociologists or anthropologists of the 19th century on incest you won't find any. Sure, there were some scattered medical reports and the like, but the practice of incest didn't really seem to pose a problem at the time
>
> (1988: 302)

With this argument there develops an ambiguity. Is Foucault suggesting that the incest taboo used to exist and kinship patterns were adhered to, as the passages in *THS* implied? Or does he mean that this is (merely) the way that the past is spoken about now, and that incest has only become cast as a social problem relatively recently, as this quotation implies?[2] This is not clarified, but it seems from his interview comments, the only other (published) place he spoke of incest in its own right, that the latter argument is the one with which he aligned himself. Certainly, the argument of *THS* still works. However the family used to be linked with incest, in discourses of this century incest is part of the discourses both 'old' and 'new', although both are actually contemporary. That is, there is a modern way of speaking which suggests that at all times *past and present* there has been a universal incest prohibition. This way of speaking about incest is contemporaneous with discourses which have the effect of sexualising the familial domain. Thus Foucault is suggesting that within the new regime incest is spoken about and constantly reaffirmed as something that belongs to the old regime. Whenever the topic is raised, incest is spoken about as prohibited and, moreover, as universally prohibited.

This clinging to the incest prohibition within the framework of a newer power is clear, Foucault argues, in the practice of psychoanalysis, the institution *par excellence* of the deployment of sexuality. It is here that 'talking sex' has been institutionalised and given the greatest credence. Yet within psychoanalysis, at its very root even, aspects more akin to the deployment of alliance are found. Despite the fact that it appears to question family relationships, and despite the part it played in taking sexuality out of family jurisdiction, psychoanalysis 'rediscovered the law of alliance, the involved workings of marriage and kinship' (1981: 113). With the Oedipus complex, incestuous desires and the operation of the incest prohibition were rediscovered at the heart of sexuality 'as the principle of its formation and the key of its intelligibility' (1981: 113).

Within psychoanalysis, the development of the notion of 'sexuality' remains tied, therefore, to the alliance network; it was guaranteed that 'one would find the parents/children relationship at the root of everyone's sexuality' (1981: 113). Without the incest taboo, which causes the parent to frustrate the child's desires, it was declared, sexuality would not be as it is. The formation of each individual's sexuality is tied to her or his familial relationships and the crucial role of both incestuous desires and the incest prohibition within those relationships. Laws of alliance were thereby incorporated into the deployment of sexuality, reappearing, now 'saturated with desire' (1981: 113), at the heart of psychoanalysis. Psychoanalysis incorporates both the agitation of the deployment of sexuality around the family's sexual activity and the necessity of the incest prohibition. Thus psychoanalysis 'made it possible to explain both the system of alliance and the regime of sexuality' (1981: 129).

The place of incest in psychoanalysis also functioned as a point of differentiation between social classes. The 'idle' woman of the upper classes was the first to take on sexuality, although eventually everyone was understood to have a sexuality (1981: 121). Foucault argues that at the end of the nineteenth century the theory of repressed sexuality compensated the bourgeoisie for the general spread of sexuality because it posited differential degrees of repression according to social class. It was held that the bourgeoisie's repression of sexuality was so deep that it was a source of constant danger to them. These dangers could be alleviated by freeing sex, allowing sex to speak. Social differentiation was therefore confirmed by the contention that there were these class differences in the intensity of repression (1981: 128–30). For the bourgeoisie, psychoanalysis was the answer, enabling liberation from this repression: within psychoanalysis individuals were encouraged to express their incestuous desires.

At the same time, there was a concern for the practice of incest amongst working-class people; their sexual desires were not repressed but acted upon. Thus the situation was such that 'at a time when incest was being hunted out as a conduct, psychoanalysis was busy revealing it as a desire and alleviating – for those who suffered from the desire – the severity which repressed it' (1981: 130).

In summary, therefore, Foucault argues that incest is a unique case within discourses of sex because it is around incest that specific aspects of the analytics of blood have kept their importance within societies which have more generally followed a trend towards an 'analytics of sexuality'. Thus he argues that when the family became a site at which discourses producing sexuality came together, and therefore became the 'home' of sexuality, the incest taboo was reaffirmed as a law that was universally obeyed. Incest seemed as though it might become the most unremarkable sexual behaviour. The constant reaffirmation of the existence of a universal incest prohibition as a fundamental law of society prevented this. Thus a tension between the two systems of power over sex was and is located around incest. Incest is both incited and denied as the family continues to form the site of the operation of the two systems. The incest taboo is momentarily lost as the family became the 'hotbed' of sexuality, and rediscovered, with particular clarity in anthropology and psychoanalytic theory, as a fundamental rule.

FEMINISM AND THE DEPLOYMENT OF SEXUALITY

Historically the feminist work on incest, stretching from the end of the last century (Jeffreys, 1985) to more recent analyses, coincides with the problematisation of incest which for Foucault signals the encroachment of the deployment of sexuality on this terrain. Moreover, feminist work is a knowledge in the sense that there is a bank of observations and a theoretical context within which they are analysed and understood. The statistics that have and are being produced due to feminist instigation of the issue of incestuous abuse can be understood as a bio-political knowledge. At first blush, therefore, it may seem that feminism is part of the deployment of sexuality. But is feminist knowledge of incest a knowledge that works within the power/knowledge networks of the deployment of sexuality? And if it does, does that mean that feminism, paradoxically, is part of a discursive incitement to incest?

Feminist work on incest, insofar as it is inescapably a 'discourse on sex', is part of the general landscape which Foucault purports to describe. But how exactly does feminist discourse relate to Foucault's arguments? In this discussion I argue that by forcing one to consider how the feminist work relates to the other discourses on incest, Foucault's arguments address questions around the status and politics of feminist knowledge. Whilst often uncomfortable, these questions enable one to build simultaneously a more reflexive account of feminist work on incest and a more robust feminist stance on certain issues – in particular, on the question of the incest taboo.

Although feminist work parallels Foucault's in its de-essentialising of sexuality, its refusal to regard sexuality as an essence that resides within the body and its insistence on the importance of social influences on sexual desires and arrangements, there are aspects of feminist work on incest which are reminiscent of Foucault's description of the mechanisms and effects of the deployment of sexuality. In particular, there are two elements of feminist work on the issue of incest which might lead one to assimilate them with discourses of the deployment of sexuality. One concerns the issue of confession, as a primary mechanism of 'talking sex'. The second concerns the disciplinary power which feminism has arguably set in place both within and around the family. I shall examine these two hallmarks of the deployment of sexuality in turn in order to see how far feminist work on incest is caught up within its web of power/knowledge relations.

The confession

Feminist knowledge of incest has resulted from listening to and restating the words of a particular group – the incest survivors – and, to a lesser extent, from collating statistics to back up the feminist case. In the previous chapter I suggested that the words of incest survivors were 'subjugated knowledges'. But in drawing them together is feminist knowledge replicating the power/knowledge strategies of the deployment of sexuality, extracting confessions upon which to base knowledge?

The confession carries with it a notion of speaking to alleviate the guilt one feels as a result of some deed. In Foucault, following Nietzsche, the guilt is always 'imposed' on the speaker by some outside morality. For example, this is the case in confessions by homosexual men in the courts of countries where homosexuality is criminal. Many women survivors of incestuous abuse (as well as rape and other forms of abuse) may feel guilty or in some way to blame because they inevitably move within those discourses which hold women at fault in sexual abuse. They may understand themselves through discourses which do not give them any way to articulate the abuse apart from a self-critical 'how could I let that happen to me?/why did I do such and such?'. A male survivor of sexual abuse may also have to confront discourses that accuse him, although in a different way from those that blame women, e.g. of not being 'man enough' to prevent it. In these ways the survivors may feel they are 'confessing'. But the 'confession' of the incest survivor is not straightforwardly a confession in Foucault's sense because it is not a confession of one's own guilty deed, even if, due to societal prejudice, the survivor may feel guilty.[3]

The difference here is similar to that which Watney (1986) draws between the confession and the assertion/affirmation of homosexuality. In his article, Watney is responding to the argument made by Minson (1981) that 'coming out' is not as radical a political strategy as it may seem because it retains the notion that homosexuality is 'about' personality and personal identity and does not challenge heterosexual ideology and power structures. Watney argues that the 'confession' of homosexuality is a personal label implying some sort of essence whereas the assertion of one's identity as 'gay' in the way that term has been formed is to assert oneself as part of a political group with a unity of interests. These interests are formed in response to the actions of others, that is, those who have categorised homosexuality as 'perverse/sick/mad/queer/contagious and so on' (Watney, 1986: 19). The 'confession' of being gay, therefore, like the 'confession' of having been incestuously abused, is not a statement about oneself, about one's own truth, but rather it is about the position in which one has been placed due to the actions of another. Foucault wished to draw attention to the way in which the process of confessing is one in which a person inscribes sexual desire as a part of the self, thereby deploying and accepting the inner truth of sexuality. Incest survivors may talk about their sexual desires within the language of the deployment of sexuality. But insofar as speaking about incestuous abuse entails speaking about sexual desires, it is not the speaker's sexuality that is at the forefront of discussion, but the abuser's.

Moreover, the feminist analyses are based not on listening to pleasure, as are the confessions to which Foucault refers, but on listening to pain. Part of the survivor's story may refer to physical pleasure, but this 'pleasure' is awkward, confusing and imprisoning: it may serve to make her feel guilty and implicated (see, e.g., Kim's story in Ward, 1984: 24–30). The survivors' accounts do not contribute to the 'great archive of the pleasures of sex' (Foucault, 1981: 63). Instead, they contribute to the feminist archives of sexual abuse carried out against women. Nor is the relationship between the woman telling her story and the woman listening comparable with that between the confessor and the court, the analysand and the therapist. Foucault states that the confession is a ritual that unfolds within a power relationship:

> One does not confess without the presence (or virtual presence) of a partner who is not simply the interlocutor but the authority who requires the confession, prescribes and appreciates it, and intervenes in order to judge, punish, forgive, console and reconcile; a ritual in which the truth is corroborated by the obstacles and resistances it has to surmount in order to be formulated.
>
> (1981: 61–2)

It is probable that women survivors speak to feminist researchers or workers within some form of power relationship. The woman listening may be considered someone who will help, or whom one has to 'please' in some way by telling the story. Of the list Foucault provides, the feminist listener may appreciate (the woman's courage) and console. However, this power relationship is not the one between analyst and analysand, nor that between accused and court, because feminist workers and researchers would try to minimise the speaker's discomfort and, in contrast to the demand for confession of every detail, respect her wishing not to talk or to tell everything. Nor is the feminist worker 'the authority' or adjudicator in her wider societal context in the same way as legal personnel can be.

Foucault suggests that the confession has become seen as an end in itself, as if it had some transformative power:

[F]inally, [confession has become] a ritual in which the expression alone, independently of its external consequences, produces intrinsic modifications in the person who articulates it.

(1981: 62)

Have feminists, with phone lines and self-help groups, fallen into what Foucault implies is a trap of presenting telling as the answer to the personal suffering caused by abuse? Most feminists would agree that simply speaking about what has happened will not have therapeutic effects. It seems that trying to combat child sexual abuse by advising children to tell someone may be ineffective, since it seems that children are already telling but they are not being effectively 'heard' (Kelly *et al.*, 1991). The effects of talking about abuse for both children and adults depend upon whether or not one is heard and heard in a supportive way. Feminist work does not regard speaking about abuse to be effective in any simple sense. Creating community between women by sharing common experiences enables one to see 'sideways' (see Chapter 3) and know that you were not the only one. Through the telling within a feminist context, the abused becomes the 'incest survivor', with the positive connotations that has in feminist discourse. But the simple rehearsing of the abuse is not an empowering act independent of such a context: the critique of the family and of societal attitudes to sexual abuse, to children, and to sexuality must receive simultaneous attention.

The Foucauldian notion of confession does raise difficult questions for feminism. Feminists are already debating many of these issues. A question mark has been placed, for example, over the ethics of getting more and more women to speak about their abuse if the only reason for their doing so is the formation of a feminist archive of accounts of sexual violence. However, this section has argued that the Foucauldian notion of confession cannot be easily assimilated to the process of knowledge formation that builds the feminist knowledge of incest, and if one takes that as one's measuring stick, feminist discourse is not part of the deployment of sexuality. But the confession is not the only tactic that signals the deployment at work. Might feminist discourse on incest be a part of the deployment in other ways?

Disciplinary power

One of the strengths of Foucault's work is his ability to illustrate that despite the stated aims of discourses of sexuality, despite the overt differences between discourses, they can work together such that their effect is a collective one. The discourses that surround sexuality and that frequently converge on the family can serve the same function. The question thus raised for feminism is how does feminist discourse operate amidst these discourses? Does feminism, in spite of itself, converge with other non-feminist discourses to produce a singular effect? In the case under discussion here, does feminist discourse join with the discursive 'noise' around the family and sex such that it may contribute both to a 'policing of the family' (Donzelot, 1979) and to the paradoxical incitement to incest as described by Foucault?

In highlighting the unsurprising nature of incestuous desires in men who live in our society feminism has arguably joined the welfarist discourses that operate as disciplinary agents around the family alerting social workers, child psychologists, teachers, etc. to the possibilities of incestuous abuse. In this way, feminism joins other, non-feminist, discourses in contributing to the operations of the deployment of sexuality around the family. Whilst this gathering of pastoral agents need not be considered a bad thing – feminists would not be perturbed at the thought that various workers are looking out for signs of incestuous abuse – what the Foucauldian argument raises is a version of the tension that has often erupted between feminism and the Left in the sense that whilst feminist work on sexual violence is radical within the terms of feminism, its effects may be considered rather reactionary in terms of the 'policing' of the family.[4] At certain points and in certain recommendations or effects, feminist work may overlap with other forms of discourse with which it otherwise has little in common. That is, feminism, and especially those feminists who get drawn, however unwillingly, into the role of 'experts' on incestuous abuse, joins a movement which surrounds and scrutinises the family, especially the more 'accessible' families where pastoral agents have established a right of surveillance, i.e. those at the poorer end of the socio-economic scale. In this way feminism has indeed joined the discursive 'noise' around sexuality and the family.

However, it is one thing to say that feminism's talk about incest joins other, non-feminist, discourses with different trajectories and different aims in focusing attention on the family and sex, and quite another to suggest that this talk may actually incite incest. The suggestion that talk about the dangers of sexuality may literally create the object of which they speak is not, however, an argument that is anathema to feminism. Indeed, Catherine MacKinnon has argued that the condemnation of sexual violence may actually incite its practice. That rape and child sexual abuse are both legally and socially condemned may, she suggests, be part of the 'excitement potential' they hold for the men contemplating sexual violence. But feminism has not generally placed itself within the realm of these disapproving discourses, although feminist voices are perhaps the most vehement in their condemnation of sexual violence. But if feminism does produce warning discourses about the family that contribute to a sexualising of the familial domain, in Foucault's sense, does this paradox render feminist discourse equivalent to those with which it is placed in the Foucauldian landscape? This would not be a corollary of Foucault's position, for *THS* was concerned with the surprising similarities arising out of *dissimilar* ways of speaking. To collapse these various discourses as if they were simply one and the same would be to lose the dynamism of the analysis, and to avoid acknowledgement of the complexities of discourses and the various configurations of which they form a part.

Whilst feminism cannot help but 'meet' other ways of speaking about sex, and whilst it is taken up by those without feminist aims, it is also fundamentally different from the discourses which Foucault seems to have in mind insofar as it contains within it a profound attack upon the institution of the family as presently constituted. Feminism does not simply 'surround' the family by raising the issue of incest, but, in attacking the very notion of a harmonious and power-free familial space, it is critical of those discourses which seek to conserve an ideal of the family. In contrast to these discourses, feminism has a deeply critical element that operates 'within' the heterosexual family ideal. Feminism draws attention to exactly that sexuality which other discourses have not, that is, the problems of 'normal' male sexuality and of 'normal' family relations. One result of the feminist discourse might be that women look out for the activities of the men around them. Thus the feminist critique sets up a 'gaze for sexuality' not only 'around' the family but 'within' the family by encouraging actors 'within' the family to operate in a similar way to those 'around' it. Foucault does suggest that the discourses of the deployment of sexuality can create divisive lines 'within' the family, e.g. between parents and children, and these discourses both institute and justify such divisions. Whilst the feminist discourse has joined this way of speaking about age/ generation divisions (something I will discuss further in Chapter 6), its radical element is that it acts to set up a gaze which challenges the gender divide. In doing so it acts as a critique of the family, and a critique of ways of speaking about the family as a unitary actor and an harmonious site. Thus feminist discourse is both within and against the discourses on the family and sex described by Foucault. It is in a state of tension with them. Within Foucault's schema it might be classed as a 'reverse discourse', a term he used to describe discourses which contain exactly this sort of tension, operating simultaneously with and against the trend of other discourses.

Redeeming feminism from the fate of being pushed into the Foucauldian mould to become 'merely' another discourse of the deployment of sexuality, however, does not mean that feminist scholars can rest back, assured of their favourable status with regard to Foucault's thesis. For feminism has become aware of the ways in which feminist discourse carries with it ambiguities and effects that are not desirable from a feminist perspective. For example, if feminism has made mothers watchful of the men in their families, it has also placed a burden on women as mothers. As with the other disciplinary agents that operate around the family, it can implicitly appeal to the mother and come to use and rely upon the mother as their agent within the family (as Donzelot [1979] describes). Women within the family may feel they have to be constantly alert for their children; they may begin to feel that they should personally watch over their children, and disallow men, either partners or other men, to be alone with their children. This role can be exploited by those agents of 'the social', making the mother responsible. Smart (1989) describes how police relied upon mothers to ensure that men accused of sexual abuse stayed away from the child(ren) during the 1987 'Cleveland affair' in Britain. In this way women become tied to their children in a protective mothering role that feminism has consistently challenged as oppressive. Thus feminism has set up a gaze within the family between women and men which, whilst radical in the sense that it draws attention to inequities within the family and the abusive behaviour that takes place within families, is also conservative in keeping women ever watchful over their children.

FEMINISM AND THE DEPLOYMENT OF ALLIANCE: INCESTUOUS DESIRES AND THE INCEST PROHIBITION

Because feminist work has concentrated on the commission of incest as a form of sexual violence, there has been a tendency to define the sociological notion of the incest taboo out of the discussion. This is not to say that there has not been feminist scholarly interest in the incest prohibition. Rubin (1975), following the work of Lévi-Strauss, argued that the incest prohibition meant that women became objects of exchange and that this 'traffic in women' functions to benefit men whilst women are in no position to benefit from their circulation.

> If it is women who are being transmitted, then it is the men who give and take them who are linked, the woman being a conduit of a relationship rather than a partner to it . . . If women are the gifts, then it is men who are the exchange partners. And it is the partners, not the presents, upon whom reciprocal exchange confers its quasi-mystical power of social linkage. The relations of such a system are such that women are in no position to realise the benefits of their own circulation. . . . Men are beneficiaries of the product of such exchanges – social organisation.
>
> (Rubin, 1975: 174)

On the whole, however, the recent feminist discussions of incest have concentrated on incest as a form of sexual violence. Taking the impetus from Foucault's discussion of incest, I want to consider the feminist position as it relates to what he termed the deployment of alliance. What would be the feminist position on the deployment of alliance, the rules governing kinship? Is the notion that there is a fundamental tension between the two deployments helpful to a feminist analysis? More specifically and more pressing for this book, what about the notion of the incest taboo, one of the fundamental rules of the deployment of alliance? What is its place in the feminist analyses? In this section I want to consider the way in which comments on the incest taboo appear at the margins of the feminist texts, and to develop these arguments into a coherent position.

Rubin suggested that the exchange of women is central to the social relations of sex and gender, thus retaining, through Lévi-Strauss, a central role for the incest prohibition which causes the social interdependence between men that constitutes social organisation. Lévi-Strauss had suggested that women were treated like language, as signs, exchanged between men, not to be misused but to be communicated (1969: 494–6). Rubin expands this into a tool for understanding sexual systems. She notes that women are 'given away' in marriage, taken in battle, sent as tributes. They are traded, bought and sold, not in the same way that some men are as slaves, but simply as women. The 'exchange in women', Rubin hypothesises, can be used as a shorthand for expressing the situation whereby men's rights to their female kin, as specified by the social relations of the kinship system, are not shared by women with regard to themselves or to their kin. The exchange of women, she argues, is a powerful concept, enabling one to place at the centre of the oppression of women not the traffic in merchandise (as Marxism had for oppression of workers) but the traffic in women. This traffic in women entails obligatory heterosexuality and the constraint of female sexuality.

Although feminist theorising of the incest taboo has given way to discussions of violence following the 'discovery' of the widespread nature of incestuous abuse in contemporary society, the notion of an incest taboo inevitably crops up in this later work. Some writers argue that the incest prohibition does not exist. Louise Armstrong argues 'a true taboo is a true deterrent. Sexual abuse of child by parent, it would seem, then, is not taboo' (1978: 9). Similarly, Rush suggests that 'there have never been firm taboos against the sexual use and abuse of children by adults, or against incest' (1980: 134). But the fact that incest occurs does not in itself invalidate the notion of an incest taboo. Although incestuous abuse may be widespread it is not widespread enough to contradict the statement that most people do not seem to commit incest. If the issue is one of numbers, of how much incest occurs, there is therefore no problem with the statement that there is a social rule that one might term 'the incest prohibition'. The fact that murders take place does not undermine the statement that in our society murder is socially prohibited.

However, despite these statements of rejection, the feminist work on incest as a whole does not reject the notion of the incest prohibition altogether. Those authors who discuss it take issue not with the statement that there is an incest taboo, but with the way the notion is presented and the assumptions contained within the concept. Herman begins with the statement that there is an universal incest taboo (Herman with Hirschman, 1981: 50), but asks why it is that father–daughter incest is not as strongly prohibited as other forms of incest. She suggests that a family structure in which there is a traditional sexual division of labour between husband and wife teaches children to hold their father in awe and to regard their mothers as subordinate. Both children turn away from their mother and value what is associated with the father; girl children learn to devalue themselves, and to fear and obey the father, whereas boy children, as well as learning that they will be the rulers of their own homes, learn 'to distrust and deny everything feminine in themselves. Their need for non-sexual physical intimacy and hunger for nurturance, expressiveness and tenderness cannot be acknowledged or gratified in the service of their development as "real little men" ' (Herman with Hirschman, 1981: 130). Herman argues that this situation creates the 'psychological conditions' favouring father–daughter incest. She suggests that in this sense the incest taboo is not 'internalised' equally by boys and girls. Women learn to be nurturant mother figures but not to impose sexual desires, whereas boys learn to expect their demands, sexual and otherwise, to be serviced by women, especially those women in their family.

Ward's (1984) argument is close to Herman's in that she too sees the incest prohibition as 'one sided' (1984: 79), and the turning away from the Mother as crucial. But Ward draws more explicitly upon the psychoanalytic concepts implicit in Herman, and particularly upon the object relations school as expressed in the work of Nancy Chodorow (1979). She argues that it is Mother–Daughter incest which is most strongly prohibited because it is the most threatening to the formation of new families and to men within the Family. Mothers have to psychically 'push' Sons away so that they may turn to their Father for gender training. Because Mothers identify with Daughters and the Daughters have to learn their gender training from the Mother, on the other hand, the Daughters are kept closer to the Mother.

This situation is potentially dangerous for the men in the family, argues Ward, because there is the possibility that the Mother will form alliances with her children, squeezing the Father out of the family. Such a move would threaten not just that particular family, but the Family as an institution and male supremacy as a whole. Thus Ward argues:

> Father–Daughter incest (rape) does *not* threaten the 'male dominated family'; nor does Son–Mother incest (rape) when the Son is an adult since he is then male dominant instead of or as well as the Father. But Mother–Son or Mother–Daughter incest would threaten existing male supremacist forms because the Father would become comparatively irrelevant to the emotional fabric which determines the relationship within the family.
>
> (1984: 188)

Ward concludes that the incest taboo, as it operates on Mothers, causing them to psychically reject their children, is a means by which male dominance is maintained. She 'gives' her Son to the Father, and keeps her Daughter at a distance. The boy represses his emotional attachment to his Mother, thereafter denying her original status for him, as well as his fear of his Father, in order to enter the world of men (patriarchy). Whilst the Mother releases her children from her sensuousness, the Father welcomes his Son into his world whilst preparing his Daughter for her 'sex object role' by treating her 'like a doll', by ignoring her, or by raping her (1984: 192).

For Ward, the incest taboo and the Family are coterminous. As such, her theory is reminiscent of Parsonian sociological functionalism, but of course it has a different trajectory. It is the Mother–Son taboo which results in the Son identifying with the Father and gives him the subconscious hatred of his Mother. Ward suggests that it is the frustrated desire together with the hatred which provide the ambivalence that is expressed in rape:

> The incest taboo *is* the family. The family is the incest taboo. (Without one the other would not exist.) ... through severance from the Mother and the subordination of women, [it is ensured that] Sons will feel hatred (misogyny) and desire (rape) for their Mothers (all women). In thus

111

creating misogynistic Sons, the incest taboo/family exists to ensure male supremacy.

(1984: 192; original emphasis)

The feminist perspective as presented in the work of Herman and Ward, therefore, does make a connection between the incest prohibition and a system of alliance. This alliance, however, is not the marriage/kinship system that revolves around blood, but a male supremacist system which revolves around power. The family system is reproduced not as an end in itself but as the site and vehicle of the male supremacist system. The incest prohibition is linked, as Rubin (1975) had linked it, with alliance between men. Ward's work also sees a 'gift' involved, but for Ward it is not women who are exchanged by men but boy children by women. In Ward's words, the most effective prohibition, the Mother–Son taboo, has the result that the Son is given to the Father by the Mother. Because of this rejection, the Sons despise and devalue their Mothers and, by extension, all women. Yet boys still feel an attraction to their first love object, the Mother/woman. As did both Freud and Parsons, Ward suggests that men are thereby encouraged to form families of their own, based upon a heterosexual union, in which they are dominant. In the world of male adulthood, they are taught the rights men have over their family. Thus the cycle begins again. Although Mother–Son or Mother–Daughter incest would disrupt this process, Father–Daughter rape does nothing to disrupt it.

Neither Herman nor Ward, therefore, relinquishes the notion of an incest prohibition, but they suggest that it does not operate in a blanket fashion across all relationships. Having said this much, however, the feminist work does not go on to reflect upon what exactly the incest taboo is, how exactly and where it operates. Foucault's work on incest provides a context within which to rethink the feminist position on the incest prohibition.

Foucault's schema appears at first to make a clear-cut division between ways of speaking about incest. On the one hand, there are those ways of speaking which place incest (as an act which is prohibited) within a system of kinship ties and blood relationships (the system of alliances). On the other, there are those which speak of incest within a context of desire and bodily pleasures (the deployment of sexuality). One might begin therefore by 'sorting' the various ways of speaking about incest into one or other category. The sociological and anthropological accounts which have focused on the incest prohibition and exogamy go one way, the psychological accounts of incest offenders as sexually perverted, the social work discourses of the dangers of overcrowding, etc., go the other. However, this division soon begins to become more complex. As Foucault suggested, psychoanalysis is situated somewhere in between, concerned both with incestuous desire and with the family structure which underlies it. Feminism, too, is 'in between' not only because there has been interest in the incest prohibition, in the work of Rubin (1975) and through feminist interest in psychoanalysis, but because the work on incestuous abuse has its emphasis both on tracing the cultural construction of incestuous desire on the part of the abuser, and on tracing a familial system in which men are dominant and incestuous abuse by an adult male is neither disruptive nor prohibited.

Perhaps then it makes sense to redraw Foucault's dual system as a continuum of ways of speaking about incest. At one extreme are those ways of speaking which deny or minimise the existence of incestuous desires and incest in any form and/or set up questions, under the symbol of blood, around the incest prohibition and kinship systems. At the other are those which, under the symbol of desire, focus on the incestuous act and ignore any connections or implications that may have for the family and social structure. What incest is 'about' therefore becomes very different at different ends of the spectrum. In between these extremes are the ways of speaking about incest which make some gesture towards the other end, as well as those, such as psychoanalysis and feminism as presently constituted, which contain aspects of each.[5]

However, Foucault's argument is stronger than offering a template for organising ways of speaking about incest, because he suggests that the power/knowledge networks of the deployment of sexuality operate around the family in such a way that they require the family as their 'anchor', for the time being at least. Insofar as they require the family, they require the discourses which create and support it in its present form. The discourses which uphold the incest taboo, inasmuch as they uphold the family, also, therefore, uphold the discourses which explore its violation. In what sense do discourses of the deployment of sexuality need the discourse of the incest taboo? Can we incorporate this idea into the feminist analyses?

The argument that the discourses of the deployment of sexuality 'need' the notion of the incest prohibition might be applied to those psychological discourses on incestuous abuse which treat the abuser as sexually perverted. Whereas feminist analyses have regarded his abuse as in some ways in accordance with male sexuality (taking a younger partner, being aggressive, perhaps experiencing his sexual desires as requiring an outlet, etc.), these (predominantly psychological) discourses speak of the abuser as 'outside' normal sexuality. The normality of the action is denied because of the relationship between the persons involved. These discourses on the perversion of the abuser, therefore, although seemingly at one extreme of the continuum (desire), can also be seen to need the other, the notion of the incest prohibition. This is because it is *the breaking of the prohibition* that justifies labelling him 'perverted' (or, perhaps, doubly perverted if the abused is young or of the 'wrong' sex). In this sense these discourses rely upon the notion of an incest prohibition, and maintain its existence in the face of evidence to the contrary.[6] In positioning the offender as perversely asocial, these psycho-medical discourses avoid the 'normality' of his behaviour and also, therefore, the feminist agenda.

The work of feminist theorist Judith Butler (1990a) is especially interesting in this context because she has discussed the incest prohibition in relation to Foucault's *THS*. Her discussion uses Foucault's arguments in an interrogation of the role of the incest prohibition. Butler shows that in Freud's account the incest prohibition is dependent upon an earlier prohibition of homosexuality, supposing as it does that the child will be subconsciously attracted to the opposite sexed parent by the time the incest prohibition does its work. (Indeed, even where Freud speaks of the child's original bisexuality, he divides the child's sexuality into a masculine and feminine part such that bisexuality means not the coexistence of heterosexuality and homosexuality, but the coincidence of two heterosexualities in one psyche: Butler, 1990a: 61.) Butler provides a Foucauldian critique of Freud's foundationalism, arguing that the notion that the child is originally bisexual, in his sense of having both a masculine and a feminine predisposition, is an assumption that his discourse creates and sustains.

Butler interprets the incest prohibition's operations as an *enforcement* of gender identity and heterosexuality. By forbidding the desired object, the taboo instigates the Oedipus complex. Butler regards the Oedipus complex as a process by which the lost (forbidden) love object is incorporated into the child's ego (or onto his/her body), as in Freud's description of melancholia, such that the object, but also the corresponding gender and homosexual desire, is 'encrypted', given a 'space' within the child's ego ideal (super-ego). Both the opposite gender and homosexuality are internalised by the ego ideal as prohibited. Thus:

> As a set of sanctions and taboos, the ego ideal regulates and determines masculine and feminine identification. Because identifications substitute for object relations, and identifications are the consequence of loss, gender identification is a kind of melancholia in which the sex of the prohibited object is internalised as a prohibition. This prohibition sanctions and regulates discrete gendered identity and the law of heterosexual desire. . . . Gender identity appears primarily to be the internalisation of a prohibition that proves to be formative of identity.
>
> (1990a: 63)

Butler is arguing that it is the incest prohibition which creates heterosexuality. In a sense, her argument might be considered in agreement with Foucault to the extent that she argues that the 'deployment' of (hetero)sexuality requires the discourse of the incest prohibition.

Having established the operations of 'the incest prohibition', Butler then moves to consider the incest prohibition as a productive law. She notes that psychoanalysis has always regarded the incest prohibition as productive in the sense that it is productive of gender identity (1990a: 76-7),[7] but her point is different. She argues that the taboo might be seen to both create and sustain the desire for the mother/father as well as ordering the 'compulsory displacement of that desire' (1990a: 76). But here she oscillates between the productivity of the incest prohibition and the productivity of the cultural child-rearing arrangements:

> The notion of an 'original' sexuality forever repressed and forbidden thus becomes a production of the law which subsequently functions as its prohibition. If the mother is the original desire, and that may well be true for a wide range of late capitalist household dwellers, then that is a

desire produced and prohibited within the terms of that
cultural context. In other words, the law which prohibits
that union is the selfsame law that invites it, and it is no
longer possible to isolate the repressive from the productive
functions of the juridical incest taboo.

(1990a: 76)

Butler seems to back away from her argument that the incest
prohibition, as a part of psychoanalytic discourse, is a law which
creates the desire that it is said to prohibit, when she refers to the
'cultural context' of mothering. She seems to resort to an
argument that accepts and 'explains' in terms of material living
conditions the incestuous desire she wished to show as produced
by the taboo. Thus Butler regards incestuous desires as produced
rather than given, although she waivers on the connection
between the incest prohibition and 'culture' as productive of
these desires. My point is that if Butler is suggesting that the
organisation of mothering produces incestuous longing, she
need not also suggest that 'the incest taboo' produces incestuous
desires.

Butler's argument seemed promising and exciting, but
ultimately her conclusions are unsatisfactory, leaving an
ambiguity around what she means by her statement that the
incest prohibition both invites and prohibits incestuous unions.
She seems to argue both that the incest prohibition creates
incestuous desires and that cultural arrangements create incestuous desires. I suggest that Butler's unsatisfactory conclusion is a
result of the fact that she remains curiously 'within' psychoanalytic discourse, placing a question mark over the production
of incestuous desires, but without doing the same for the incest
prohibition, and considering the incest taboo only in relation to
the infant's desire (with the adult's desire assumed to be relatively
unproblematic). Indeed, she seems to accept the concept of the
incest taboo, stating that her purpose is to stress that the incest
taboo is not merely prohibitive but productive, in its production
of both gender and sexuality: 'In other words, not only does the
taboo forbid and dictate sexuality in certain forms, but it
inadvertently produces a variety of substitute desires and
identities that are in no sense constrained in advance' (Butler,
1990a: 76). In short, the incest taboo is only interrogated insofar
as Butler contests its repressive nature.

I want to take a further step 'outside' psychoanalytic discourse in order to think about the status of both concepts: 'incestuous desires' and 'the incest prohibition'. Butler begins to question the former, but for feminist work on incestuous abuse, the issue of the incest prohibition needs to be interrogated as well. I want to question the Truth of the incest prohibition in relation to Foucault's arguments on the continuum of ways of speaking about incest, and in relation to feminist arguments about incestuous abuse, desire and the incest prohibition.

My point of departure is the observation that many ways of speaking about the incest prohibition, including the theories on its origins, sociological accounts of its function, and psychological accounts of incestuous abuse, assume that there is such a thing as 'the incest prohibition'. Much anthropological work has begun to question the usefulness of this label, arguing that perhaps not all writers on the incest prohibition are discussing the same range of phenomena (Goody, 1971). My argument, however, is not that the incest prohibition varies over cultures such that the term 'the incest prohibition' homogenises very different cultural systems. Rather, I am arguing that the very notion of an incest prohibition is highly problematic. Its existence and status are frequently taken for granted and assumed to be a fact of societies. Theories of the origin of the incest prohibition have frequently pre-supposed that which they are trying to explain, sociological theories of kinship assume that the incest prohibition exists (and, furthermore, that it is efficient) and psychological theories around the perpetrator assume that something called 'the incest prohibition' has been traversed.

What happens if we do not presuppose the existence of the taboo, if, instead, we regard it as a discursive construction, a Truth that exists only to the extent that we speak about it?

It is of course a truism to say that the incest prohibition exists only insofar as we speak about it: there is no object 'the incest prohibition' that we can pick up and handle. But this rather simple point reveals, quite uncontroversially, that 'the incest prohibition' is in the first instance a *descriptive* term that purports to describe the workings of a social rule. It describes certain forms of behaviour or lack of behaviour – incest avoidance – as well as certain attitudes – the 'horror of incest' – and is a label for these observations. The point I am making here is that initially one has to understand 'the incest prohibition' not as what leads to incest avoidance and attitudes toward incest so much as a description of these phenomena. If it is a descriptive term it cannot then be posited as the cause of what it describes. Later, however, I will suggest that a causal role, differently formulated, can be retained for 'the incest prohibition'.

The second point is that many ways of speaking about incest also presuppose incestuous desires that have to be controlled. Psychoanalytic discourse is clearly both the reason and the prime example here. Incestuous desires on the part of children toward their parents is a fundamental tenet of psychoanalytic theory. Indeed, where incestuous desires have been denied, as in Westermarck's (1921) thesis that the incest prohibition was a moral rule which followed rather than caused the avoidance of sexual relations between kin, the theory was widely dismissed. Westermarck suggested that there is a lack of erotic feelings between those who have lived closely together since childhood, and that this aversion then became custom and was only subsequently expressed in the form of a moral prohibition. At the time he was criticised with the argument: if incest was avoided, why would there need to be a prohibition? Such an argument illustrates how the incest prohibition was accepted as a fact prior to its explanation, my first point, above.

Westermarck's reception suggests that the existence of incestuous desires was widely accepted. Among followers of Freud, at least, this would have been the case. Freud argued that Westermarck's hypothesis left no room for the emotions of the Oedipus complex and should be abandoned (Freud, quoted in Arens, 1986: 71). Thus Freud takes his theory to be based upon indisputable facts which Westermarck's theory cannot explain. To this, Westermarck replied that he saw no evidence of repressed desires to commit incest, that this was a 'supposition' rather than an 'unearthed fact' (in Arens, 1986: 71). From my different angle, I want to argue that the incestuous desires of psychoanalytic theory are indeed suppositions, 'facts' produced by psychoanalytic discourse. The existence of incestuous wishes on the part of children and the existence of the incest prohibition are essential components – constructions – of psychoanalytic theorising.

When incestuous abuse or behaviour does occur, it has frequently been understood in ways that do not challenge the existence of the incest prohibition. Incest has been regarded as sexually deviant, as the expression of a perverted sexual desire (e.g. Gebhard *et al.*, 1965; Barbaree and Marshall, 1989). In fact, the occurrence of incest has been regarded as evidence both of incestuous desires and, since relatively few cases occur, the strength of the incest prohibition (Lindzey, 1967).[8] Even in some feminist writings on incestuous abuse, the status of the incest prohibition goes unchallenged.

I would argue instead that 'the incest prohibition' is created and sustained by anthropological, sociological, psychological, psychoanalytic, legal and 'common sense' discourses at both ends of Foucault's continuum. It has become a Truth which is unchallenged and upon which several theories and writings rely. This was Foucault's point when he argued that 'the great interdiction against incest is an invention of the intellectuals' (1988: 302). 'Beyond' the incest prohibition, furthermore, there is frequently (although not always) the notion of 'incestuous desires' which are also, I suggest, theoretical constructions that have taken on the status of Truth. But where does this leave one? Are there no incestuous desires and is there no incest prohibition?

Feminist analyses have already made a move away from previous understandings of 'the incest prohibition', refusing the incest prohibition a place in their theoretical arguments. That is, incestuous abuse is understood not as the traversing of a line – licit/illicit – but as actually informed by accepted discourses that are in themselves *nothing to do with incest* (but are to do with sexuality, power and the family). In this, feminist analyses have made a direct challenge to the notion of the incest prohibition. However, as discussed above, the incest prohibition, in its various modified forms, still remains in several feminist texts. If one suspends all belief in both an incest prohibition and incestuous desires, adopting a Foucauldian attitude of scepticism, how can one then recast the feminist arguments?

A fundamental argument in feminist analysis is that within the family power is exercised and knowledge is distributed in unequal ways. Lines of age and gender, whilst not necessarily fixing the exercise of power, are lines across which power is negotiated with certain predictability.[9] The term 'incestuous desires', however, does not distinguish between these different positions within the family. It does not distinguish between men and women, nor between adults and children. What happens to notions of incestuous desires and 'the incest prohibition' when one considers the different positions within the family?

For the child, psychoanalysis posits incestuous desires toward the parent(s) which the parents then frustrate in deference to an incest prohibition. Butler (1990a), *inter alia*, has suggested that the child's desire for the mother may be the result of social structures which mean that in late capitalist societies, at least, children tend to spend their infanthood with their mothers. This caretaker then becomes the only security the child has known. However, in what sense are these desires sexual? What counts as sexual? Psychoanalyst Alice Miller has criticised the tradition in which she was trained, arguing that although the child may have a desire for 'love, care, attention, and tenderness' (1985: 121) from the adults around him or her, and s/he may have a 'healthy and intense curiosity' (1985: 122), it is doubtful that s/he has an image of sexual stimulation or intercourse in mind. A desire to be a sexual partner is not what attracts him/her to the adult. She writes: 'I understand the concept of "infantile sexuality" as a pedagogical way of thinking that overlooks the actual imbalance in power' (1985: 124). The term 'incestuous desires' conflates the child's sensual desire and desire to receive attention with the sexual desires of adulthood. Thus one can argue that the child's desire for the parent/caretaker does not amount to 'incestuous desire' if incestuous is taken to mean sexual in the sense of sexual stimulation or intercourse.

It is the Father's incestuous desires which have been the focus of most feminist work on incestuous abuse. As I discussed in Chapter 3, in feminist analyses the Father is understood as positioned within discourses of sexuality and the family that are in themselves unconcerned with incestuous abuse but which render the abuse 'intelligible'. From a feminist perspective, the Father's incestuous desires are understood as informed and condoned by accepted, indeed traditional, discourses. This argument does not mean that all Fathers have incestuous desires; the discourses which inform the abusing Father's behaviour do not *have to* produce abusing Fathers. The complexity of discourses by which individuals 'turn themselves into subjects' and the many paths by which an individual negotiates his or her way through those discourses means that any such conclusion would be simplistic. Nevertheless, the feminist analyses have convincingly argued that it is the Father's position, a potential

120

position, that any 'incitement to incest' surrounds. The Father's incestuous desires are culturally informed at the intersection of a number of discourses.

On closer inspection it is clear that these desires are not necessarily *incestuous*, in two senses. First, they are desires that are focused on family members, most frequently on girl children, not because they are family members but for other reasons such as the fact that these people are the closest to hand, because the Father has some authority over these people, because he may feel he has some 'right' to them, etc. In this way the feminist analyses have taken the Father's abuse 'outside' the family. In other words, to say they are incestuous is to label this desire in a way that sees desire as always already tied to the object of attraction, or, more accurately, to the relationship between the desiring agent and the object of desire; but that relationship may be more a feature of social organisation (e.g. of living accommodation) than a characteristic of the *desire*. Secondly, the Father's 'incestuous desires' may not be incestuous because they may not be about sexual gratification. Some feminist analyses argue that incestuous abuse is about power in this sense, although most now argue that power and male sexuality are so entwined that incestuous abuse is both sexual and about power.

When men do not abuse their children, is this evidence of an incest prohibition? From the perspective being argued here, it is not; or, at least, it may not always be. Men's understanding of their sexuality, masculinity, role in the family, fatherhood, are informed by discourses of the culture in which they live. But since the position of the abusing Father is only ever a potential subject position, one way of 'negotiating' the discourses on male sexuality and the family, it is not inevitable that all men will fill this position, and there are of course many men who do not feel 'incestuous desires'. If this is the case, some men have no need for the intervention of an incest prohibition. That is, their 'avoidance' of incest is *not a response* to an incest taboo. The point is that the notion that an incest prohibition is 'at work' on every individual parent's behaviour presupposes the existence of incestuous desires: the incest prohibition is either traversed or obeyed. However, if incestuous abuse is not 'about' the breaking of the incest prohibition, feminist analysis can theorise the occurrence of incestuous behaviour *as well as its avoidance* without need to posit the existence of 'an incest prohibition'.

It is not contradictory to add that 'the prohibition of incest' as a discursive phenomenon may still be relevant both when men do not abuse members of their family (or do not engage in incestuous romantic relationships, for that matter) *and* when they do. For these behaviours *may* be in response to an incest prohibition; that the prohibition is a discursive construction does not mean that it cannot inform incest avoidance. When aware of their incestuous desires, men may not act upon them in deference to an incest prohibition. I would argue that the incest prohibition functions by making people consider the reaction their behaviour would receive. The imagined reaction may be somebody's reaction in particular, people's reaction in general, or the law's response. Finkelhor (1984) and Russell (1984) have argued that there are certain factors that may prevent sexual abuse occurring. The incest prohibition may be one of these factors in the sense that the actor poses himself the question 'what would people say?' (This anticipated response may also prevent consensual incest, although in this case the couple have the powerful discourse of romantic love within which to understand and present their behaviour.) When such a thought is entertained and the act is not taken as a result, then one can meaningfully speak of 'incest avoidance'. On the other hand, MacKinnon's (1982) argument that the prohibition or illegality of acts can be 'part of their excitement potential' suggests that the 'prohibition of incest' as a discursive phenomenon may also be involved in the *commission* of incestuous abuse. This is a form of Butler's argument that the incest prohibition creates that which it is said to prohibit. If MacKinnon is correct, 'the incest prohibition' acts as an incitement in the form that the abuser asks himself 'what would people say if they knew I was doing this/had done that?' The thought of their negative response may excite him, make him feel powerful, or, in Cameron and Fraser's (1987) analysis, make him feel 'transcendent' because he feels he no longer needs to obey the rules of society. If this is correct, it is by the anticipation of others' talk that the incest prohibition functions. The incest taboo is a way of talking that can have a role in the avoidance of incest but also in the commission of incest; at the same time as it prevents, it can play a part in the production of the act it forbids. It is the possibility for talk (the condemnation of the act) to which the actor responds, whether or not he commits the act. Indeed, to all intents and purposes, the response of others constitutes 'the incest taboo'. This argument is not altogether new in sociological discussion. In 1967 an article in the *American Journal of Sociology* argued that 'publicly approved criticism' is the 'empirical manifestation of incest taboos' (Young, 1967: 600). However, I would wish to avoid the implication that there is something (what could this be?) that was the 'real' incest taboo underneath the manifestation of this condemnation.

The retention of the notion of 'the incest taboo' in feminist work has been principally to explain the *mother's* behaviour. Again, however, to explain the mother's behaviour as an act of deference to an incest prohibition is to presuppose incestuous desires. What mothers do may be described as 'incest avoidance', but the very suggestion that incest is avoided implies that incestuous desires were felt and that they were refused. The feminist analyses suggest that fewer mothers than fathers sexually abuse their children for a variety of reasons: because they are the carers of children, they tend to be closer to children, to know them as individuals with their own desires, to respect those desires, because female sexuality is not focused on younger people, nor on being demanding and predatory. In short, they tend to lead lives in which they relate to children as subjects rather than as objects. It is not that women sexually abusing children is impossible: this is clearly not the case from the (very small numbers) of women who have done so. But in terms of the construction of female sexuality, motherhood and the family, it is more surprising. In short, incestuous behaviour on the part of the mother is not discursively incited in the same way that it is for men. To state that they 'avoid incest' assumes the refusal of incestuous desires, and to claim that the Mother–Son taboo is 'stronger' is to fail to interrogate the presumptions of the incest taboo and incestuous desires. Yet the feminist arguments suggest that mothers avoid incest for reasons other than in response to an incest taboo. So why retain such a notion to 'explain' her behaviour?

In summary, therefore, one can argue that the notion of the incest taboo as a Truth which stands rigidly in place in each and everybody's lives needs to be interrogated. Perhaps 'the incest prohibition' needs to be understood instead as a discursive construction, one of some stature within several discourses. Via Butler (1990a) and Foucault (1981), I have suggested that the incest prohibition exists only to the extent that we talk about it, or, more accurately, the incest prohibition exists only to the extent that we talk about incest as prohibited, undesirable behaviour. To understand the incest prohibition as a discursive phenomenon in this way is not to deny that it exists nor even to deny that it can function as a deterrent. The fact that incest is considered immoral, criminal and perverted, and that social institutions reiterate and operate around this understanding, is not to be dismissed: these attitudes, constituting the substance of 'the incest taboo', may well play a powerful part in preventing incestuous acts. As a discursive construction, however, its effects are neither rigid nor straightforward. Although it may 'work', therefore, and it may actually be involved when incest is avoided, maybe 'the incest prohibition' can also be *irrelevant* to the avoidance of incest. It may *describe* that avoidance, but the idea that everyone who avoids incest has done so in *response* to an incest taboo fails to question whether the taboo was necessary to produce that 'incest avoidance'. That is, was the desire there in the first place? Might s/he have avoided incest for reasons other than the incest taboo?

Once it is accepted that sexuality and sexual desires are constructed, 'incestuous desires' cannot be presumed to exist in every individual. Groups of people (men, women, children) are differently positioned in discourses of sexuality and in discourses of the family, making suspect the notion of incestuous desires as a foundational Truth. The incest taboo's 'attempt' to encourage incest avoidance, therefore, is unnecessary where individuals do not have those desires. Even when incest does occur, one does not have to retain a conception of incestuous desires 'behind' it; a Father's desires may be directed at family members without being intrinsically 'incestuous' at all. Moreover, the incest prohibition can be also be implicated in the *production* of incest; it can be understood as producing incest as it attempts to repress it. If it is correct that the flouting of rules is exciting and provides a feeling of empowerment, as MacKinnon (1989) and Cameron and Fraser (1987) suggest, an awareness of the prohibition, the wrongness of incest, may also be implicated in the production of incest, both abusive and non-abusive. It would be over-dramatic to claim that the incest taboo never operates to prevent incest; however, the success of the incest taboo is not predetermined.

Once the incest prohibition is understood as a Truth sustained by a cluster of theories and practices, it makes sense to interrogate the processes involved in its continued currency. In the next chapter I turn to British criminal law on incest, where the incest taboo is instituted in the form of 'thou shalt not', in order to do just this.

5

WHAT'S THE PROBLEM?
The construction and criminalisation of incest

In the stark form of 'thou shalt not' the incest prohibition is enshrined in both English and Scots criminal law. Thus criminal law on incest appears to be a model example of juridico-discursive power, laying out the forbidden and threatening punishment if the command is disobeyed. However, in this chapter I argue that this bald statement of prohibition rests upon several different ways of constructing incest as a problem: what masquerades as a simple restatement of a prohibition entails the mobilisation of ways of speaking which are less juridicial and more akin to the power/knowledge networks of the deployment of sexuality. In order to argue this point, the chapter investigates the parliamentary debates which shaped the current legislation on incest.

The law of incest that now exists in Britain was put into place in 1908 in the case of English law and in 1986 in Scots law. In this chapter I want to consider both laws, and I am therefore dealing with parliamentary debates from two different periods. The first set of debates are those that took place around the criminalisation of incest in English law at the beginning of this century. Incest had not previously been a crime in English law.[1] It had been dealt with by the Church up until 1857, when the removal of power from the Church left incest neither an ecclesiastical nor a criminal offence (Wolfram, 1983).[2] There were several unsuccessful attempts to pass the Bill criminalising incest (in 1899, 1903 and 1907). The debates I have studied are those when the Bill was discussed at length: those of 1903, when the Bill was unsuccessful, and of 1908, when it was passed. The 1908 Act was later incorporated into the 1956 Sexual Offences Act. The second set of debates took place in the 1980s and dealt with the revision of Scots law. In Scotland incest has been criminal since 1567 but this Act was not updated until the 1986 Incest and Related Offences Act. The Act was still in old Scots, and criminalised the 'abhominabill, vile and fylthie lust of incest' with reference to the relevant chapter of Leviticus. It was argued that new legislation was necessary because each time the Act was used, there was debate around which relationships were included within its rather imprecise terms and courts had had to consult copies of the Bible in use in 1567 from the National Library. Those involved in the drafting and debating of what was to become the 1986 Act had, therefore, to start from scratch in their decisions about what form the crime of incest should take in Scotland. The Scottish Law Commission researched and drafted the Bill which formed the basis of the eventual Act. With the parliamentary debates of the 1980s, therefore, I have included the Scottish Law Commission's work (the 1980 Memorandum and 1981 Report).[3]

The crime of incest in both English and Scots criminal law refers to sexual intercourse between a man and a woman who are related to one another as indicated in the legislation. There are differences between the relationships criminalised by the Scots and English legislation. Whilst the relationships within the 'nuclear family' are criminalised in both, the Scots legislation is more comprehensive, including more relationships than the English. In England, for example, the uncle/niece, aunt/nephew relationships are not punishable as incest, whereas they are in Scotland. The Scots legislation also has clauses referring to step-children and 'intercourse of person in a position of trust with child under 16'. In both countries incest is constituted solely by the act of penetration of the vagina by the penis. In both, consent is no defence (for fuller details see Appendix I).

In considering these debates, I do not want to get drawn into a discussion about their timing or causation.[4] Instead, the focus is on *how* incest is spoken about and my exploration therefore takes the form of a discourse analysis. The wish to approach the study of law in this way arises from a wish, as Goodrich has suggested, to 'analyse law from outside legal culture . . . in terms, most simply, of its semantic functioning (regularities) and of its history, its relation to and representation of, power' (1987: 132). Such a methodological approach has been detailed by Potter and Wetherell (1987), whose work has been influenced by, *inter alia*,

Foucault and theories of the constructive power of discourse. They introduce the notion of an 'interpretive repertoire', which at its most general can be thought of as a way of talking and of understanding something. In this case, I am looking for the interpretive repertoires that the speakers in the parliamentary debates use to talk about and understand incest. Although Potter and Wetherell note that there is no 'cook book' for identifying repertoires within the discourse, one searches for phrases and arguments which suggest a certain way of understanding.

For example, the suggestion that incest is 'against God's will' or is a moral offence which transgresses some code of behaviour set down by a higher order, either God or Nature or the more abstract 'moral society', appears in the parliamentary debates in both periods. Thus in the 1903 debate one speaker refers to incest as 'an offence not only against morality and decency but against every instinct of human nature' (Lord Davey, Lords, 16.7.1903) and in the 1980s debates a speaker refers to a common abhorrence of incest:

> We might today – most of us – express our repugnance at the idea of sexual relations between close blood relations in language somewhat different from that of the legislators of 1567. However, I should have thought that the repugnance is surely at least as strongly and widely felt.
> (Lord Wilson of Longside, 9.12.1985, Lords)

Perhaps more interesting, however, is the way in which speakers construct incest as a wrong with reference to what one might term 'knowledges' in the sense that there is a body of writing and a set of 'experts' which accompany the assertions. My focus is on how these knowledges of incest are articulated in the debates and the ways in which they inform the crime of incest as it appears on the statute books. I argue that what seems a clear form of juridico-discursive power has been informed not only by the statements of prohibition which it mimics, but also by the 'rational' arguments of bio-political knowledge. In light of the arguments of Chapter 4, the incest prohibition is (re)created as a Truth which relies upon the deployment of sexuality for its continued articulation. It is in this sense an unstable legal construction.

Incest has become an issue to which several knowledges are addressed and the debates around incest draw upon several different justifications for the criminalisation. Each knowledge constructs incest as a particular kind of wrong, placing particular demands on the terms of the legislation. The result is that during the debates the object under discussion – 'incest' – shifts its meaning and its terms of reference according to the knowledge by which its 'wrong' is being asserted. Emerging from this battle of knowledges is the legal category 'incest', which, whilst dependent upon the knowledges that have shaped it, is not reliant upon any one of those knowledges to define its parameters. The argument, therefore, is that the legal prohibition of incest is the result of several different ways of speaking about incest, ones which span the continuum of ways of speaking from those that focus on the incest prohibition and kinship networks to those that focus on sexual dangers.[5]

In particular, I want to highlight how the debates construct incest as a *specific* crime: that is, how the different knowledges suggest that there is a specific wrong of incest such that it cannot be dealt with by other legislation (e.g. rape and sexual offence laws) but requires separate legislation. In doing so I am making an argument about the process of law creation. Carol Smart (1984; 1989) has argued that that the law itself is a form of knowledge which has the power to disqualify other accounts of social reality. As I discussed in Chapter 1, Smart's work uses Foucault's work in order to make arguments about the interaction between different forms of knowledge at the site of law. In my analysis of the parliamentary debates on incest, I take a step 'backwards' from the court room situation in order to consider the process of law creation, a process in which law does not yet have a knowledge from which it can 'disqualify' other knowledges, but is, instead, the site at which various knowledges, each presenting its 'truth' of incest, meet and map out a space for incest as a specific crime.

I have divided the knowledges articulated in these debates into three sections. First, I consider the construction of incest as a problem of inbreeding; secondly, I consider those knowledges that construct incest as wrong because it causes harm to a living individual; and thirdly, I consider those knowledges that construct incest as a threat to the institution of the family. In tracing the articulation of these different knowledges in the debates I shall not be assessing the relative truth of the knowledges, but indicating how they produce different arguments about the wrong of incest, each with an attendant image of what and whom incest involves. These images conflict as well as coincide. Ultimately, this discursive battle of knowledges is silenced and denied when the legislation is presented and understood as a coherent response to a singular problem. This is therefore an investigation of how the law's Truth is constructed at the level of the statute.

INCEST AS A PROBLEM OF HEALTH: THE INBREEDING ARGUMENT

One of the ways in which incest is presented in the debates is as a problem of health. According to this knowledge of incest, what is wrong with incest is the potentially deleterious effects of inbreeding. The health in question is that of the potential offspring, and, on occasion, this becomes the health of the nation. Although this problematisation of incest was not voiced in 1903, in 1908 there were references to the risks of incest by four separate speakers. Here are two of those four:

> Mr. MacLean of Bath said . . . he had known of instances producing no less than three or four children of weak intellect, idiots and imbeciles. The cases were of the most grave kind.
>
> (26.6.1908, Commons)

> In a certain number of crimes of a similar character it might be argued that it would be desirable not to take steps with regard to them, because they effect nobody but those immediately concerned; but your Lordships will see that that is not the case with regard to crimes of this character, and that there are, as a result of intercourse between the various people mentioned in the Bill, offspring on whom the punishment chiefly falls.
>
> (The Lord Steward, Earl Beauchamp, 2.12.1908, Lords)[6]

In the 1980s, the inbreeding argument is still alive and well, clearly articulated in the debates on the revision of the Scottish legislation. In the Scottish Law Commission's Memorandum (1980) and Report (1981) 'genetic reasons for prohibiting incest' are given as one of the four main arguments for retaining the crime of incest.[7] The Memorandum states:

[I]ntercourse between certain persons should be prohibited because the offspring are more liable to exhibit physical and mental abnormalities.

(1980: 22)

The studies upon which the Commission draw are ones which have observed and 'measured' children born to related parents, seeking to find quantifiable differences in terms of health but also in terms of mental ability and general 'intelligence' (the studies include Adams and Neal, 1967; Seemanova, 1971). These researchers are thereby constructed as the experts on incest, the ones who have produced scientific truths of incest. The importance of the inbreeding argument in the debates on the 1986 Act is underlined when the Commission consider whether the crime of incest need remain a specific offence in criminal law, or whether other areas of law, such as rape or sexual offences laws, would adequately deal with the wrong of incest. They state:

In our view, to have no such provision would be to take less than proper account of genetic considerations.

(1980: 59)

Several commentators have argued that on its own the inbreeding argument is insufficient justification for criminalising incest (e.g. Wasoff, 1980; Mason, 1981). Amongst several objections to the inbreeding argument as the basis of law is the argument that legislation based on such an objection to incest would logically have to disregard cases where there was no danger of conception, e.g. because one or both parties was unable to conceive for medical reasons, for reasons of health or age (too young or too old). This limits the criminality of the act to specific groups (the fertile) and specific times (during fertile years, possibly even fertile days). It further limits the criminality to the consequences of the act, suggesting that if no pregnancy follows, the act itself was not wrong. It suggests there is nothing intrinsically wrong with incestuous intercourse, but the possible consequences are such that it should be criminalised. Yet despite the arguments that have questioned the inbreeding argument, it seems to be repeatedly rehearsed when incest is discussed.

My question with regard to the inbreeding arguments is not how important the inbreeding argument was in the passage of the Bill. Nor do I ask whether it is relevant or even accurate (in the past or now). My question is instead: how does the inbreeding argument function in the parliamentary debates? How does it inform the meaning of the term 'incest', and how does it relate to the process of mapping out a place for incest as a specific crime? The presence of this knowledge in the debates brings with it some important correlatives that construct a particular image of incest.

First, it constructs and relies upon an image of incest as sexual intercourse between a man and a fertile woman, and, therefore, as heterosexual and between adults (in the sense of being able to conceive). When the 1981 Report considers including 'homosexual' offences, it is the inbreeding argument that is used to argue that they should not be included. Secondly, it constructs incest as only between people related by blood ('full' or 'half' blood). Step-father/step-daughter incest, for example, is not included in its image of incest. Thirdly, the 'victim' of incest is depicted as the potential offspring. Finally and importantly, incest becomes a specific wrong. It is constructed as wrong for reasons that other behaviours are not. The wrong of incest is something other than the wrong of rape, for example, and therefore needs to be separated from rape. It is in this sense that the place of incest is being discursively 'mapped out'. The inbreeding problematisation of incest gives incest a specificity, backed up by scientific fact, that disallows its collapse into other categories of offence.

Despite the importance given to the understanding of incest as a problem of health-risk for the potential offspring in the Law Commission's work, in the parliamentary debates of 1985 and 1986 it is hardly articulated, possibly because the debates tend to centre on how to include step-children in the Bill (where genetic considerations would be out of place) with blood relatives presented as unproblematic, as 'obviously' included. There is however, an interesting exchange in the Standing Committee in which the continuing importance of the genetic argument in the justification for criminalising incest is highlighted. When the first speaker constructs incest as a problem of non-consent, this understanding of the wrong of incest is challenged. The genetic argument is then offered (as well as linking incest to the cohesion of the family, to which I shall return), acting in this way as the guarantee of the specificity of incest:

Mr Fairbairn: ... It seems that it is only when there is abuse rather than consent that one should generally expect a prosecution to arise. ...

Mr Maxton:　　　. . . In the latter part of his speech, the hon. and learned Member . . . began to talk about the law having to deal with abuse in terms of incest. He began to sound as if he were saying that incest is all right provided both sides consent, and that we should prosecute only when there is abuse. That is not the view of the law. . . .

Mr Fairbairn:　　. . . If the law is to be sensible, it will not prosecute wrongs because they are nameless wrongs, but wrongs which do harm. The prosecution must always bear in mind the wrong that one is trying to strike at, which either is a threat to the cohesion of the family or would lead to genetic deterioration [sic]. . . .

(11.6.1986)

Thus, when challenged on his understanding of incest as wrong because it involves abuse, the Member reverts or defers to the genetic argument. The inadequacy of this problematisation is pointed out in the reply:

Mr Maxton:　　. . . I give the example of a man of 40 who marries early and has a daughter when he is 19. His wife dies and he is a widower; he has a daughter now of 21. If he sleeps with her for the first time and there is consent between them, does the hon. and learned gentleman say that that is legitimate because he may have had a vasectomy and therefore is not capable of procreation and there is no danger to the species?

(11.6.1986)[8]

This exchange also illustrates the way that different constructions of the problem of incest shift the meaning of incest and the image of the incest situation that accompanies it.

Reading these debates from a Foucauldian perspective, one might see the references to offspring as part of the movement he has described whereby

governments perceived that they were dealing not simply with subjects or even with a 'people', but with a 'population' with its specific phenomena and its peculiar variables: birth

133

and death rates, life expectancy, fertility, state of health, frequency of illnesses, patterns of diet and habitation.

(Foucault, 1981: 25)

At the heart of this economic and political problem of population, Foucault continues, was sex. In order to 'know' and keep in touch with the population, it became necessary to analyse

the birthrate, the age of marriage, the legitimate and illegitimate births, the precocity and frequency of sexual relations, the ways of making them fertile or sterile, the effects of unmarried life or of the prohibitions.

(1981: 24–5)

The references to the effects of inbreeding, therefore, could be connected to the operations of a style of governing, one that watched over the health of the nation through the study of its life and its sex. Whilst these debates do not give us any real evidence that this was new, it does seem that the inbreeding argument has all the aspects that Foucault associates with this new form of government, with its use of what he termed 'bio-power'. This form of power is bi-polar. At one end there are these techniques directed toward the population as a whole. At the other end there are disciplinary techniques, directed toward the individual body.

The studies of inbreeding, both those that were around at the time of the English debates and the more recent studies quoted by the Scottish Law Commission, display these disciplinary techniques. Nineteenth-century studies looked at close-breeding communities, measuring their bodies and recording the results in a 'scientific' mode, seeking any differences that could be attributed to the inbreeding.

At Boyndie, in Banffshire, and Rathen, in Aberdeenshire, the fishermen are a very closely bred community, the former somewhat shorter and lighter than the landsmen, and their heads are not quite so big.

(Huth, 1875: 150, reporting a study by Beddoe)

The measuring and observing did not always support the inbreeding hypothesis, however:

[In Burnmouth and Ross, Berwickshire,] there was no case of a lame, deformed, blind, dumb or paralytic person to be heard of; and in the school, which was twice visited, and

where nearly all the children were assembled, no strumous
sores were found, nor were any of the children puny, pale
or languid, but on the contrary, merry and active.
(Huth, 1875: 148, reporting a study by Mitchell)

Similarly, the later studies on which the debates of the 1980s
draw investigate the children of incestuous unions, using more
'sophisticated' measures such as IQ tests, and more complex hypo-
theses drawn from genetics, but with the same general hypothesis at
work and with the same disciplinary gaze that seeks out quantifiable
differences to report and present as knowledge, as scientific truths.

INCEST AS A PROBLEM OF ABUSE: THE PROTECTIONIST, PSYCHOLOGICAL AND FEMINIST ARGUMENTS

In this section I consider those arguments that see incest as
wrong because of an immediate abuse of one or more of the
parties involved. It is a harm against a living individual or
individuals.[9] This understanding of what incest is 'about' is one
that clearly conflicts with the inbreeding argument, and, indeed,
one that would render the inbreeding argument irrelevant, since
whether or not there is a danger to a further individual (the
offspring) in no way changes the fact of the immediate harm
done to the individual concerned. This would be the wrong that
feminists see in incest, for example, although it is not the case that
whenever incest is constructed as wrong in this way it reflects a
feminist knowledge of incest. I have identified three ways in
which incest is spoken about as an immediate harm (these are not
necessarily mutually exclusive): in arguments that equate incest
with child abuse; in arguments that stress the psychological
effects of incest; and in feminist arguments that stress the gender
differential in incest. I shall deal with these in turn.

Child abuse

The 1903 Bill, in its original form, constructed an image of incest
as involving intercourse between an older male and a younger
female insofar as the criminalised relations for a man were
daughter, grand-daughter and sister, and for a woman they were
father, grand-father and brother.[10]

In the 1908 debates, too, incest was constructed as an attack upon children by an adult man. The expertise and the knowledge of the National Society for the Prevention of Cruelty to Children were brought into the debate in order to illustrate that cases of incest do occur (the Lord Bishop of St Albans, 2.12.1908, Lords). These agents of a Foucauldian 'pastoral power' not only provided evidence that incest did occur but framed it within their particular concern for children. A telegram from the Lord Chief Justice read out in the 1908 Lords debates also depicted incest as an assault by a man upon a younger female:

> You can state that I support the Bill. I have received and sent to the Home Secretary presentments of grand juries pointing out the urgent necessity for an amendment of the law, in consequence of the frequency of assaults by fathers on their daughters.
>
> (Read out by the Lord Bishop of St Albans, 2.12.1908)

Such a construction of incest is not always used in favour of the Bill, however, since it was also argued that an Incest Bill was not necessary because most cases could be dealt with under the Cruelty to Children Acts or under the Criminal Law Amendment Act (the Earl of Crewe, 2.12.1908, Lords).

The notion that incest is a form of child abuse from which children need protection is also present in the 1980s debates. The Scottish Law Commission's Memorandum suggests that punishment must be justified 'in terms of society's present ends. We would place high among those ends the strengthening of the fabric of the family, and the protection of its members *especially children* from injury and molestation' (1980: 57; emphasis added). Speaking of raising the age to which step-children are included as a 'related offence' from 16 to 21, one of the Lords argues: 'This amendment is to add to the protection which the young person, the step-child, would have in the family' (Lord Morton of Shuna, 28.1.1986, Lords).

The psychological impact

In the 1980s debates, however, a possibly more dominant understanding of incest is that which draws upon psychological knowledge. In the Scottish Law Commission's (1980)

Memorandum, there is a chapter entitled 'The Psychological Effects of Incest', and this understanding of the wrong of incest is given much space in that document. Here the wrong of incest is the psychological harm caused to the female incest survivor. The studies which report the psychological effects of incestuous abuse involve a disciplinary gaze, and often one which positions the abuse as a disruption of 'normal development'. In doing so there are assumptions being made about what counts as 'normal development', particularly sexual development. For example, the Memorandum states that the female survivor of incest is endangered by the 'premature development of sexuality without adequate means of coping with the sexual tension' (1980: 37). Drawing on further scientific studies, it suggests she is then prone to seek outlets for her inner turmoil by way of anti-social behaviour and drug use.[11]

These psychological studies tend to uphold the reified notion of the incest prohibition of which I spoke in Chapter 4. Thus one study, speaking of the female survivor, states 'once the incest barrier is broken, it is easier to advance to other forms of deviant behaviour, particularly promiscuous sexual behaviour' (Benward and Densen-Gerber, 1975, quoted in Scottish Law Commission, 1980: 37). Another states that 'the prohibition broken, the behaviour tends to continue with the girl becoming more and more acquiescent until a relationship almost comparable to that of a marriage is established' (Allen, quoted in Scottish Law Commission, 1980: 35). Thus the incest prohibition is set up as a gateway which, once passed, takes one into a world of deviancy and illusions. Allen suggests furthermore that the girl enjoys this relationship until it becomes known to the family, at which point she feels guilty and 'plays the part of the victim of the relationship' (Scottish Law Commission, 1980: 35).

In the psychological problematisation, moreover, incest is seen as a problem that will lead to the female survivor becoming a 'problem' for society (she will become 'anti-social'). In this way, interestingly, the psychological knowledge of incest constructs incest as a threat to future generations in the same way that the inbreeding argument does. Drawing on a study of incest as a 'causative factor' in anti-social behaviour (Benward and Densen-Gerber, 1975), it is argued in the Memorandum that 'the result could well be a second generation of inadequate persons who will produce subsequent generations of neglected children unless we develop tools for prevention, detection and treatment of these families and their children' (1980: 36).

Moreover, the psychological knowledge often brings with it implicit theories about the causes of incest, further depictions of what incest is 'about'. In the Memorandum, and in the later Report (1981), one way in which incest becomes spoken about is as a problem of family functioning whereby certain families are set up as dysfunctional. The Scottish Law Commission's (1980) Memorandum quotes at length from a study by Maisch (1972). This work saw incest as a result of 'family disorganisation' which had preceded it. Each member of the family, but particularly the parents, is depicted as contributing in some way to the incest. The disorganisation of one family is described with reference to

> the negative influence of the husband on the shaping of the marriage and the family in the first place, a similar negative influence on the part of the wife; violence and irascibility often associated with drinking on the part of the father; and promiscuity, an unsettled way of life, drinking and drug-taking on the part of the wife together with her physical illness often leading to absence from the home. The daughters of these parents evinced symptoms of disturbed personality development either in the form of psycho-somatic symptoms, dissociality (as e.g. truancy, running away from home, frequent lying, undesirable sexual relations) or neuroses and other behavioural disturbances (e.g. anxiety symptoms such as fear of death, claustrophobia and suicidal tendencies) or depression.
>
> (1980: 32–3)

The feminist critique of such psychological assertions has highlighted the way in which the notion that the particular families in which incest occurs are dysfunctional provides a way of taking the responsibility off the abuser, as well as very often blaming the mother as in the above description, e.g. listing the mother's illness and absence as evidence of her contribution to 'disorganisation'. There is a psychologisation of incest that depicts the family as in some way 'abnormal'. Simultaneously there is a normalisation strategy within this type of knowledge, since there is an implicit model of organisation to which this disorganisation is contrasted. But it is the normal Family itself that feminist knowledge places at the centre of the problem.

The feminist perspective

The feminist knowledge of incest is not incompatible with aspects of the previous two understandings of the wrong of incest. However, some aspects of them are clearly quite different, especially where the implicit causes in the psychological knowledges quoted by the Law Commission are concerned.

Whilst it seems that feminist, along with social purity, movements were important in getting the Incest Bill on the agenda at the time, in the early debates a feminist understanding of incest is not explicitly articulated. In the 1980s debates, however, again a time of feminist activity around the issue of incest, there are some comments that present a feminist knowledge. Incest is compared with rape and the issue of consent is problematised by the Commission:

> The quality of the offence is often indistinguishable from that of rape. While consent may not be completely absent, it is difficult to differentiate between threats, duress, acquiescence and willingness in a situation where the man is in authority over the child.
>
> (1980: 69)

In the same way an amendment to raise the age to which a step-child is included within the crime of incest challenges the concept of consent (although the comparison this speaker makes with unrelated rape would need to be challenged as well):

> [I]t is an open question whether one can usefully talk in terms of a daughter's or son's consent, particularly if one takes into account the fact that the young girl in an incest situation is subject to a completely different set of conditions regarding defence, tolerance and participation from the child or maturing girl who meets a completely unrelated adult aggressor.
>
> (Scottish Law Commission, 1981,
> quoted by Lord Morton of Shuna, 28.1.1981, Lords)

There is only one speaker, a woman, who constructs her argument from an unmistakably feminist knowledge of incest. She tells the House:

> I have been forced to be interested because of the increasing and, in many ways, welcome discussion about incest, which until fairly recently has been swept under the carpet. We

should all welcome the fact that now both men and women are beginning to discuss these problems, which are particularly difficult for the girl or young woman involved in what amounts to violence against her by a member of her family . . .

Many women of all ages have told me of the pressures on them from their fathers, stepfathers or, in some cases, their elder brothers to develop a relationship. It can start at an early age when the young girl does not know what is happening, is frightened, and knows something is wrong but does not know what.

(Ms Richardson, 4.7.1986, Commons)

Tracing the construction of incest as a harm against a living individual, therefore, takes one into a consideration of the child protection, the psychological and the feminist arguments about what is wrong with incest. The 1903 Bill did seem to reflect an understanding of incest as involving an older male and a younger female, but the debates do not reveal a feminist knowledge of incest. In the early debates, the construction of incest as a harm against a living individual is represented on this parliamentary level by the protectionist argument. In the work of the Scottish Law Commission in the 1980s the psychological arguments are accorded the most space of these three constructions of incest as an immediate harm. It is not until the 1986 Commons debates that a feminist knowledge seems to be explicitly drawn upon and incest is constructed as violence against young women and children within the family (Ms Richardson, 4.7.1986, Commons).

In a broad sense, these three understandings of the wrong of incest are compatible. But they do differ in the image they construct of incest. The victim of incest in the psychological studies, for example, is sometimes the family as a whole, as opposed to one individual. The protection arguments stress the age difference, the fact that it is the category 'children' who are at risk. This would not be compatible with a feminist perspective which, whilst it does consider the fact that the abused is very often 'a child' as important as the balance of power relations, lays more emphasis upon the wrong of incest as sexual abuse related to the gendered power dynamics of a male-dominated society that depicts women and children as possessions of the male.

HAPPY FAMILIES: INCEST AS A PROBLEM OF THE FAMILY

The third major way in which incest is constructed as a problem is the construction of incest as a problem of the family. I have already mentioned the way in which incest is spoken of as the result of a disorganised family system in some of the psychological studies. In this section, however, I want to look at the way incest is constructed as wrong because it threatens the *institution* of the family.

In the early debates, although the family was spoken about as under threat, it was the criminalisation of incest that was set up as the danger to the family, not the practice of incest itself.

> [P]oor people were forced to live together, men and women often in the same room, and it was easy enough for anybody to make accusations which could not be disproved against parties who were totally innocent. They would make family life impossible if they passed such legislation. They would make it impossible for members of a family to live at home without running the risk of terrible accusations being brought against them.
>
> (Mr Lupton, 26.6.1908, Commons; see also
> Mr Staveley-Hill, 26.6.1908, Commons)

In the 1980s debates, by contrast, the protection of the family is a recurrent understanding of the purpose of the crime of incest. In the Memorandum the authors note that 'there is a core of theory associating the prohibition [of incest] with the need to preserve the family'. Echoing a sociological functionalist line of argument (see, e.g., Parsons, 1954), they state: '[the family] is the fundamental unit of all larger social groups and the principal means of preparing the child to participate as a mature adult in the life of his community' (1980: 3). In order to preserve the institution of the family, the Memorandum depicts the criminalisation of incest as 'controlling the potentially disruptive cross-sex attractions and rivalries engendered within the family' (1980: 3).

It is interesting to note the way in which the assumptions of this knowledge are overlaid upon the law of incest. In these arguments around preserving the family it is cross-sex attractions that are held to be the danger. This may be because of the

141

influence of Freud on functionalism through the work of Talcott Parsons, since Freud's Oedipus complex was based upon the assumption that unconscious attractions are always to the opposite sexed parent. The Parsonian knowledge sets up the potential attractions in the family as only cross-sex, and thereby provides a justification for the fact that the crime of incest involves only male/female vaginal intercourse. This is also true of the inbreeding argument, which relies upon incest as being male/female. These knowledges did not *cause* the crime to be so limited because they would be *post hoc* justifications. Nevertheless, they construct the image that 'fits' the crime.

The construction of incest as wrong because it threatens the institution of the family is seen again in the Report's argument that relationships of affinity can and should be removed from the crime of incest because, *inter alia*,

> there is less risk of harm to the solidarity of the family since in-laws rarely form part of the typical family household in contemporary Scottish society.

(1981: 19)

Similarly, in the Standing Committee the exclusion of relationships of affinity is presented as a response to the changing family structure in Scotland, with the implication that they no longer form a part of 'the Family' which the Bill seeks to preserve:

> [T]he genetic argument is not there because the parties are not related by blood, . . . there are other provisions to protect children, and . . . *increasingly in Scotland there is not the same family structure as in times past.*

(Mr Wallace, 11.6.1986; emphasis added)

The inclusion of the adopted child/adoptive parent relationship as incest in the 1986 Act might also be interpreted as relying on a problematisation of incest as a threat to the Family, because it disregards genetic links within it and places more emphasis on social links.[12] In the Standing Committee the way in which the inclusion of adopted children is presented constructs this understanding of the wrong of incest:

> Admittedly there is no blood tie, but because of the other factors which society deemed important, and *the reason why the law of incest should exist – principally the question of trust and*

the family bond – it was thought that the adopted relationship
was such that it should come within the crime of incest.

(Mr Wallace, 11.6.1986; emphasis added)

When the Lords debate what age limit to place on the
inclusion of step-children, one speaker suggests that he understands the criminalisation of incest to protect marriage, and by
extension the family. He also constructs an image of incest as
cross-sex and consensual:

It is fairly obvious that a 16-year or 17-year old young lady
may be attractive to and attracted by a stepfather, and it
appears astonishing to remove any sanction and so permit
such a relationship which would be wholly destructive of the
marriage between the stepfather and his wife.

(Lord Morton of Shuna, 9.12.1985)

The understanding of incest as wrong because it threatens the
family sometimes seems to equate incest with adultery, and as
disruptive to kinship (alliance) systems. For example, in the
Standing Committee, one speaker says:

Is it not right to act on the first principle that if a man
chooses to marry the woman, he should not sleep with the
[her] daughter or any one else?

(Mr Forsyth, 11.6.1986)

The discrepancy between the incest and the marriage laws
becomes a problem for this speaker as it becomes clear that the
proposed legislation would not criminalise sexual intercourse
between a step-parent and a step-child over the age of 16 but that
they would not be allowed to marry until the younger party is 21
years old. This, he suggests, will lead to social problems. First, it
would lead to more 'one-parent families' (Mr Walker, 4.7.1986,
Commons). Secondly, in a way that echoes the inbreeding
arguments' construction of the offspring as the victim of incest,
he suggests that the child of the step-daughter and father would
be made miserable.

More important . . . are the children who are likely to result
from such a relationship. Does any one really believe that
children conceived in this way would not at least have a real
prospect of becoming what is known as problem children –
another concern for our modern society? . . . Does any one

believe that bastards conceived between a step-father and a step-daughter aged 16, 17 or 18 can hope to become anything other than, at best, a curiosity to other children and members of the community where they live? . . . At school they will be given, I have no doubt, hideous and horrendous names.

(Mr Walker, 4.7.1986, Commons)

In these ways, therefore, incest is constructed as a problem because of the wrong it causes the institution of the family. Criminalising incest, in turn, becomes a way of safeguarding the family and by extension, the society as a whole. This problematisation maps out a space for incest as a specific crime because the law becomes understood as part of the incest prohibition, which is constructed in turn as the basis of the family structure on which society is built. The crime of incest has therefore to reflect the family structure that it wishes to protect (hence, for example, the relationships of affinity are not included because they are not considered part of that family structure).

DISCUSSION

The occurrence of incest is never denied in these debates. How widespread it is, where it occurs and the question of whether it is increasing or decreasing is another matter. During the early debates, there are those who are concerned that 'cases do very often occur' (the Earl of Donoughmore, 16.7.1903, Lords) and that legislation must be brought in to deal with these cases. However, there are also suggestions that the criminalisation of incest would be superfluous, since incest could be dealt with under other laws (the Earl of Crewe, 2.12.1908, Lords). Others (Mr Lupton and Mr Staveley-Hill, 26.6.1908, Commons) argue that criminalising incest could be dangerous, leading to the imprisonment of innocent people or, 'by methods of administration, to other and graver evils' (Mr Rawlinson, 26.6.1908, Commons) or even to 'the danger of something that never entered the heads of people being put there by proceedings of this kind' (Earl Russell, 2.12.1908, Lords). Finally, it is argued that legislation may be unnecessary, because incest is fading away. This last argument constructs incest as a primitive behaviour that 'civilising influences' will cure:

There was no suggestion that this offence was on the increase; indeed, it was far less known now than it was twenty or thirty years ago in parts of England. . . . Was there the slightest reason to doubt that the spread of education and of civilising influences was doing away with this evil?

(Mr Rawlinson, 26.6.1908, Commons)

In the later debates there is no suggestion that criminalising incest is dangerous in itself; indeed the debates in the Houses are taken up with discussions around how to include step-children, with the criminalisation of intercourse between blood relatives unquestioned. Nor is it suggested that incest is fading away. Rather, it is suggested that the knowledge we have of incest cases is 'the tip of the iceberg'. This perspective is backed up with reference to the views of 'experts':

The noble Lord, Lord Morton, referred to the tip of the iceberg theory. This has been a theory which has been widely held. I recall when involved in cases of incest many years ago hearing this view expressed by many social workers, medical men and others.

(Lord Wilson of Langside, 9.12.1985, Lords)

In the 1980s debates, this perspective seems to be the consensus. Incest has been established as a social problem, one that needs to be uncovered, studied and debated; its place within the operations of bio-power seems firmly established. One speaker declares:

I find it [incest] so horrendous and horrible that I want all aspects of it properly and fully debated.

(Mr Walker, 4.7.1986, Commons)

The 1980s debates also contrast with the earlier debates on the question of where incest takes place. In the 1903 debates some speakers attempted to enclose incest within 'boundaries', making incest a problem of geography, spatially located. Incest is related to the 'rural districts' (Colonel Lockwood, 5.3.1903, Commons), as well as to the bigger cities (Earl of Donoughmore, 16.7.1903, Lords). This geographical placing of incest can be regarded as understanding incest, on the one hand, as a primitive behaviour, as have many academic analyses of the incest prohibition, and, on the other, as an urban phenomenon associated with modernisation processes that brought the working classes to the cities where housing was inadequate, as had the 1888 Royal Commission on the Housing of the Working Classes. The assertions of the speakers in the debates were not purely speculative on the part of the individuals involved insofar as they drew upon these bio-political knowledges, knowledges which involved the exercise of power in their formation, especially disciplinary techniques of surveillance and examination. On the one hand, academic work, such as that quoted by Huth (1875), presented certain isolated communities as the ones in which incest was practised. On the other, official and charitable investigations associated incest with housing and city life. The Royal Commission on Housing carried out extensive investigations of a clearly disciplinary nature, calling 'witnesses' from the spectrum of disciplinary agencies (e.g. medics, social reformers, charity workers) who revealed the practice of incest. Thus, in these early debates, incest is constructed as a geographical problem being either a subcultural practice of isolated communities or another sexual danger in the urban life of the working classes.

In the mid-1980s it is clear that incest has secured a place as a social problem to be aired and discussed. It is no longer placed within boundaries. Indeed, this type of boundary-making is explicitly rejected. But talk about incest takes many forms, and although the later debates indicate that people are discussing incest, the knowledges being constructed and articulated are certainly diverse. The debates on incest span Foucault's continuum. Sometimes incest is located within discourses on sexual danger, e.g. the early references to the possibility of people copying an incest case or the remarks made around the issue of consent that see the family as a dangerous place:

> I understand that it is extremely difficult to prove whether or not consent was given, demanded or accepted. . . . We have to reach a decision. . . . All this happens within the family home *where there is a real danger of abuse*.
> (Mr Walker, 4.7.1986, Commons; emphasis added)

At other times the discussions are pulled into issues of alliance. The following speaker locates the debates on incest clearly at the 'alliance' end of the continuum.

I am no lawyer, but merely a politician who believes that

there is a duty on this place to do everything it can to strengthen the institution of the family. . . . I am worried about passing legislation which seems to suggest that it is perfectly alright to sleep with one's step-daughter provided she is over the age of 16 and gives her consent, but that one cannot marry her until she is 21 . . . how can it be right for our law to allow an act which could result in the procreation of children but not allow that act to take place within the institution of marriage?

(Mr Forsyth, 11.6.1986)

CONCLUSION

In this chapter I have discussed three of the most important ways in which incest has been constructed as a problem in these parliamentary debates: as a problem of health, as a problem of harm to a living individual (which I divided into three), and as a threat to the institution of the family. These are three understandings of the wrong of incest that are recurrent in the debates. Behind the bald criminalisation of incest found in criminal law, therefore, there is a web of interweaving knowledges and ways of understanding incest as a problem. In a Foucauldian schema these understandings frequently (but not always) belong to the deployment of sexuality in that they are part of the will to know about sex. They are comprised of studies that seek to find out about incestuous sex, to establish a knowledge about it.[13]

It is not surprising that the image of whom incest involves changes as the various knowledges construct the 'incest' to which their comments are addressed. Sometimes speakers construct an image of incest as a consensual act between adults, as the inbreeding arguments often do; sometimes as an act of abuse between an adult and child; sometimes as the behaviour of members of a psychologically abnormal family. In the main incest is spoken about as if it involves an adult male and a younger female. This does not signal a feminist victory, however, for although it is compatible with a feminist understanding of incest, this image does not always reflect an understanding of incest as a gender issue, nor one of child sexual abuse. Indeed, who counts as a child is an issue which is debated in the sense that the speakers do not agree on the age to which step-children should be included in the Scots legislation.

British law on incest has been built up from these several different knowledges of incest. None of these is the sole knowledge upon which the law is based. The differences between the various problematisations of incest in the debates are not, in fact, addressed as differences. Their coexistence in the debates, and the fundamentally different positions that they may represent or suggest, is not acknowledged. Indeed, the coalition of several knowledges has probably been instrumental in the process of law creation, with the different knowledges building and contributing to the forming of a law which may not have been so created if only one knowledge were articulated or if the discrepancies were probed too deeply. Thus where the inbreeding argument breaks down, the family argument can be brought in to protect the place of incest in the criminal law. In this way the law is reliant upon several knowledges. Indeed, the law's position, in both English and Scots law, might be described as eclectic, taking aspects of various knowledges in building its position. In this, I am echoing Smart (1984; 1989), who has suggested that the law has to be understood as complex and contradictory, with little of the autonomy or coherence it purports to have.[14]

The legal discourse on incest has been a meeting place for relations of power/knowledge. Disciplinary techniques of power have been operating in the formation of the knowledges that have then met at the site of law. But the analysis of these debates illustrates that the legal discourse is not impenetrable. The challenge of the feminist knowledge on incest can and has been represented in the process of law creation. It has provided another way of conceptualising incest which has received space in the discussions. Yet the 'discursive battle' that took place between the various knowledges of incest established none as victor, but, rather, produced a further Truth, a powerful truth that subsequent legal procedures have taken as their point of departure.

In short, this chapter has been a study of the 'problematisation' of incest. Foucault explained that this concept does not mean the 'representation of a pre-existing object, nor the creation by discourse of an object that doesn't exist', but, as mentioned in Chapter 2, it refers to the practices that introduce something 'into the play of true or false and constitutes it as an object of thought' (1988: 257). The debates reveal how incest has become an 'object of thought' within several different discourses – medical, social welfare, feminist and so on – that have different understandings of what incest is 'about' and that have produced different sorts of knowledges of incest. When the different knowledges meet, as they do in these debates, the very parameters of what constitutes the 'truth' about incest are continually attacked and reconstituted.

The debates are in a sense simply a site at which these various truths of incest are rehearsed. But the law on incest is more than this, as I suggested at the beginning of this chapter, since it is itself in the juridico-discursive mode. Although some of the speakers in the debates suggest that they must respond to 'the incest prohibition', they are not merely responding to it but are continuing it; the law makes a discursive command that incest is prohibited. As such, it forms a part, and an important and powerful part, of the incest prohibition.

6

MAKING MONSTERS,
LOCATING SEX
Foucault and feminism in debate

In Chapter 2 I suggested that the practical programme to which
Foucault's work leads involves a questioning of discursive
categories that surround us. His question would be something
like: 'how does this way of speaking about things constrain us,
repeat patterns of power, perpetuate related relations of power,
contain lines of weakness where resistance might challenge the
habitual nature of our thought?' In this chapter I want to
consider two debates in which Foucault took part in which he
asks these sorts of questions and which are particularly relevant
here because the comments he makes set him in conversation
with feminist thought. Whilst neither of the debates is about
incest *per se*, they are both pertinent since they concern adult–
child sex and rape respectively.[1] In the first debate the issue
under scrutiny is the nature of the childhood sexuality that laws
protect and the consequent creation of 'monsters' defined by
their desire for children. In the second, the issue is whether or
not rape should be treated as a sex crime or as a crime of violence.
The questions Foucault raises are difficult and even impossible.
Such an interlocutor is bound to expose contradictions and
important unresolved problems. But whilst feminism cannot
answer these queries satisfactorily, neither does Foucault. In
exploring the confrontation between Foucault and feminist
thought, the chapter argues that whilst in both cases one can
agree on some level with Foucault the theorist, and one can
admire Foucault the question-master, one can also disagree with
the 'ethico-political' decisions he offers.

MAKING MONSTERS? THE CASE OF
ADULT–CHILD SEX

In 1978 Foucault took part in a debate in which, together with Guy Hocquenghem and Jean Danet, he argued that sexual relations between adults and children should not be restricted by the law (Foucault, 1988). Collectively they had made a submission to the Penal Code in France calling for the removal of the laws which forbid the incitement of minors to 'debauchery' and criminalise relations between minors and adults. In the debate they centre their arguments on the notion of 'childhood', suggesting that these laws construct and rely upon an historically specific notion of childhood which has links with a whole network of disciplinary power/knowledge relations. Guy Hocquenhem suggests that whilst there has been a trend toward a liberal approach to sexuality, there has been a simultaneous resurgence of conservative opinion which appeals to a certain notion of childhood:

> These new arguments are essentially about childhood, that is to say, about the exploitation of popular sentiment and its spontaneous horror of anything that links sex with the child.
>
> (In Foucault, 1988: 273)

Because public opinion and the opinion of the 'psy' professionals refuse the very possibility of consensual sexual relations between an adult and a child, children are constructed, they argue, as a particular population, not *without* a sexuality but with a fragile sexuality. Thus whilst psychiatric knowledge now holds that children do have a sexuality – '[they say that] we can't go back to those old notions of children being pure' (Foucault, 1988: 276) – it now constructs a *specific* sexuality for the child. Foucault describes it as follows:

> This territory of the child is a territory with its own geography that the adult must not enter. It is a virgin territory, sexual territory, of course, but territory that must preserve its virginity.
>
> (1988: 276)

By suggesting, moreover, that sexual relations between children and adults are always, by definition, traumatising, psychiatry effectively robs the child of the chance to say that s/he did consent: 'what takes place with the intervention of psychiatrists in court is a manipulation of the child's consent, a manipulation of their words' (Danet, in Foucault, 1988: 274). Psychiatric knowledge is regarded by the contributors to this debate as the real villain of the piece. Psychiatrists have it both ways, Foucault argues, since it is denied that the child has the ability to consent, whilst it is also asserted that if s/he did, help is needed to protect the child from his/her desires.

Foucault suggests that the case of adult–child sex is indicative of a new form of penal system in relation to sexuality, one 'whose function is not so much to punish offences against these general laws concerning decency, as to protect populations and parts of populations regarded as particularly vulnerable' (1988: 276). His argument, therefore, is that there is a discursive line being drawn between adult and child in the realm of sexuality, with children constructed as a 'high risk', vulnerable segment of the population. The relation that is constructed between adult and child sexuality is, furthermore, 'extremely questionable' (1988: 277).

In parallel with this construction of the forbidden and fragile sexual territory of the child is the construction of the 'dangerous individual' who trespasses there. Danet suggests that the law's purpose is to seek out 'the pervert'; and legislators have been determined to start by 'tracking him down in the most dangerous institutions, the institutions at risk, among the populations at risk' (in Foucault, 1988: 275). Teachers have been an obvious target. The argument being made here is therefore tracing a move similar to that highlighted in *THS* (Foucault, 1981). A category of persons has been defined through their sexual inclinations/desires, a discursive move from acts to roles. By surrounding this person with legal, psychiatric and sociological knowledge 'an entirely new type of criminal' (Hocquenhem, in Foucault, 1988: 278) is simultaneously described and constructed. He is defined, moreover, by his desires.

The overall tendency of today is indisputably not only to fabricate a type of crime that is quite simply the erotic or sensual relationship between a child and an adult, but also, since this may be isolated in the form of a crime, to create a certain category of the population defined by the fact that it tends to indulge in those pleasures. There then exists a particular category of pervert . . . of monsters whose aim in life is to practice sex with children.

(Hocquenhem in Foucault, 1988: 277)

In this debate Foucault and the others are making explicit a manouevre that is only ever implicit in Foucault's books, that is, the move from theory to policy, from descriptive geneaology to prescriptive (or moral) stance. The form of the argument is a familiar Foucauldian one. The debaters argue that legal discourse actually produces what seems a natural division (adult sexuality/child sexuality) and maintains that division by statute and with the support of a cluster of disciplinary knowledges (of which psychiatry is the foremost). Thus Foucault places a question mark over the naturalness of the division so produced, the suggestion being that the paternalistic attitude expressed in law is not a response to facts of sexual development, but an expression of opinion. These laws relate to 'crime[s] of opinion' (Hocquenhem in Foucault, 1988: 278), reproducing moral notions around sexuality and divisions between populations (adult/child, paedophile/'normal'). In doing so it allows control of those populations. The argument is reminiscent of the argument of *THS* (1981) insofar as it discussed the creation of certain personages (homosexual, hysterical female, etc.), including the sexuality of the child.[2] But whilst the theoretical argument is similar, the overt practical suggestions made in the debate (and in the submission to the Penal Code) are to be found nowhere in *THS*. If one wishes to argue that there is a normative or critical postion there, it has to be sought out in the slightest of phrases. For the most part, Foucault seems to rely on the normative position of his readers, who are left to ponder the pros and cons of the various discursive constructions, and whether or not life was better before the discursive divide. In the debate, by contrast, Foucault and the others are clearly taking up their position.

The theoretical argument that legal discourse is part of a policing of a boundary between adult and child sexuality is interesting and, as a broad outline, convincing; there is no straightforward and observable division between adult and children's sexuality and any attempt to delineate one would be foolhardy. But the policy suggestion made by the debaters immediately opens up room for critique.

Foucault and the others object to the laws through an appeal to a form of freedom, using what appears to be a 'no constraints' type of rallying cry. In this appeal to change the law and legal practice in the name of the rights of both the child and the adult, Foucault seems to forget his well known scepticism of this notion of rights and this notion of 'no restraints' as freedom. Perhaps he believes this would be a favourable negotiation of the power networks within which we move. But in *THS* he had argued that power does not have one source, but is fragmented and mobile, web-like. The deployment of sexuality cannot be traced to one institution or form of knowledge; it is an effect of many. In the debate, on the other hand, Foucault seems to be speaking as if the law were solely responsible for the suspect division and as if removing the law would remove it. In this reification of the law as the sole cause of the division, he seems to revert almost to the juridico-discursive understanding of power. It seems more plausible, and more 'Foucauldian', to argue that if the law were removed, there would be other discourses and practices (psychiatry is a case in point) that could continue to maintain the divisions that the debaters address. These other discourses do not rely upon the law for their continued articulation.

This might not pose a problem for Foucault, who might argue that the existence of these other discourses does not prevent us from challenging one brick in the wall. But the point is that *because* of these other sites of construction the collapse following the removal of the one brick is going to bring with it rather worrying consequences.

Whilst one might agree on a theoretical level that the division between adult and child sexuality is 'merely' discursive, that discussions addressing children and sexuality are more frequently than not imbued with reactionary morality, that paedophilia is a category that has been created discursively and that depicts 'paedophiles' as 'monsters', the proposal offered by Foucault *et al.* does not provide the answer. The proposal to remove the legislation is worrying, especially for the feminist reader reading it in the context of feminist activism around child sexual abuse. In the ten years between the debate and its publication in English, feminism has put child sexual abuse onto the agenda and has managed to get it taken seriously by the law and the media. There are still battles to be fought, especially in the legal arena.

Foucault suggested that 'the ethico-political choice we have to make every day is to determine which is the main danger' (1986a: 343). I shall argue that the choice we make in this case should not be to support the type of move Foucault *et al.* are proposing. I argue that debaters' suggestions would in all probability lead to a worsening of the legal situation. Thus although the suggestions made in this debate make a radical 'Foucauldian' point (a theoretical point that might promote thought on the part of the legislators), they may not be progressive suggestions in practice. Indeed, they would, in some important senses, be conservative moves.

Foucault and the others argue that they are not talking about violent incidents. Hocquenhem states that

> we took great care to speak exclusively of *attentat à la pudeur sans violence* (an indecent act not involving violence) and *incitation de mineur a la débauche* (incitement of a minor to commit an indecent act). We were extremely careful not to touch on the question of rape, which is totally different.
>
> (In Foucault, 1988: 283)

In contrast, feminism *has* tended to see the question of adult–child sex as more or less the problem of rape. This is because the way child sexual abuse came to be 'heard' in feminist campaigns was through its similarities to rape. As a consequence of this, the problem has been assimilated into feminist discourse as a problem of sexual violence. Thus feminist analyses have not really addressed the notion of consent nor discussed consensual adult–child relations (and consensual incest). These questions have not been on the feminist agenda. But if they were placed there, how would feminist analyses deal with these issues?

Feminist theorising has moved away from the concept of violence that Hocquenhem employs, one that is easily distinguishable from consensual relations. Brownmiller's (1975) early feminist work on rape argued that men and women need to make explicit their consent each time they enter sexual relations since for too long women's consent has been assumed and non-consent has been ignored. Later feminist work, however, has argued that all heterosexual encounters entail a violation of women. MacKinnon (1982) has argued that forced sex is paradigmatic of gender relations. Through such arguments the notion of consent has become highly problematised in feminist work. How can a woman really consent to a sexual encounter with a man when she is never in any real position to refuse? Her context, especially if she is married and economically dependent, means that she can only 'consent'. In short, the notion of consent is in danger of disappearing from feminist work as women's own understanding of consent is elided (Vega, 1988).

If consent is meaningless between men and women, it is even more clearly meaningless between adults and children. For these reasons, one is often faced with the argument that it simply does not make sense to talk about consent in debates about child sexual abuse. The argument is that in terms of the social, economic and cultural positions occupied the child is going to begin from an unequal position. The 'choice' of whether to consent or not is going to be taken within a qualitatively different context, not because of some natural dividing line between the adult and child, but because of the positions the two inhabit in the contemporary world. This seems to be the stance adopted by Finkelhor, who is quoted approvingly by feminist Emily Driver:

> adult–child sex is wrong because the fundamental conditions of consent cannot prevail in the relationship between an adult and a child . . . even if someone could demonstrate many cases where children enjoyed such experiences and were not harmed by them, one could still argue that it was wrong because children could not consent. The wrong here is not contingent upon proof of a harmful outcome.
>
> (Driver, 1989: 5)

But this leads to the same problem as the debates on rape. Are two consenting individuals ever in a position of pure equality? Are we saying that children can *never* truly consent because of their social position? Is this a protective stance or the continued regulation of certain boundaries? Which is 'better'? If we want to argue, as does Vega (1988), that feminism needs to put women's own understanding of consent back into theorising about rape in order to make some practical sense of the feminist debates, does that also mean that in parallel we have to accept a notion of consent for cases involving children?

This firing of questions at oneself is, I think, exactly what Foucault would have wanted to prompt. But how does this questioning really help us? Does doubting a rigid feminist stance make us warm to the Foucauldian?

156

The immediate fear of feminists listening to the debate would of course be that decriminalising adult–child relations would mean that instances of child sexual abuse would go unpunished because the offender would have the opportunity to argue that the child was consenting. The solution cannot be as simple as 'listening' to the child, as Foucault seems to suggest: 'the child must be trusted to say whether or not he was subjected to violence' (Foucault, 1988: 284). Jean Danet suggests how present attitudes to the two crimes differ. He argues:

> When we say that the problem of consent is quite central in matters concerned with pedophilia, we are not, of course, saying that consent is always there. But – and this is where one may separate the attitude of the law with regard to rape and with regard to pedophilia – with regard to rape, judges consider that there is a presumption of consent on the part of the women and that the opposite has to be demonstrated. Whereas where pedophilia is concerned, it's the opposite. It's considered that there is a presumption of non-consent, a presumption of violence, even in a case . . . in which the charge is that of *attentat à la pudeur sans violence* (an indecent act not involving violence). . . . We must certainly see how the system of proof is manipulated in opposite ways in the case of rape of a woman and in the case of indecent assault of a minor.
>
> (In Foucault, 1988: 283–4)

The debaters are here concerned with only one one of these 'manipulations' – that children are assumed never to consent. They are suggesting that children are never given the conditions 'in which they can say what they feel' (Foucault, 1988: 285) and that law should 'listen to what the child says and give it a certain credence' (Hocquenhem in Foucault, 1988: 285). Whilst the concern that children's perspectives are ignored is an admirable one, the effect of abolishing this piece of legislation in isolation would have the effect of putting the child in the witness stand, in the same legal position as the woman in the rape trial. The danger with such a move is that because of the difficulty of proving non-consent, such a trial would become like the rape trial with the cross-examination employing the same tactics as those used in an adult rape trial, where the woman is called a liar, her sexual conduct is scrutinised, her behaviour judged (see, e.g., Adler, 1987).

Moreover, it seems that with the British law on statutory rape, where such tactics should be irrelevant and where establishing the occurrence of intercourse and the age of the girl is all that should be discussed, the suggestion that the child consented or that the accused had reason to believe s/he was consenting is *already* made in trials *despite* their legal irrelevance (Burman, 1989). Thus the presumption that children do not consent may not even be the situation in practice as the debaters believe. Indeed, historically it seems children have more frequently been accused of consenting when they did not than vice versa.

Foucault and the others contend that the rights of the individual are being disregarded by the state's deployment of a particular sexual morality. The right that they seem to guard is the right to express one's sexual desire as one wishes regardless of one's age. Whilst Foucault and Hocquenhem seem to somehow dismiss the notion of consent because it is simply a contractual notion (Foucault, 1988: 285), they themselves are making an argument that depends crucially upon it. In effect, the debaters are wishing to incorporate children into the framework of contract theory by which the law approaches sexual relations by arguing that children can give consent. In effect, they wish to argue that children are individuals and should be treated in the same way as adults. But this 'individual' is an abstract notion that of course never exists in reality. Whilst the law may speak about individuals, the practice of law is with men and women, girls and boys. My position parallels that of Carole Pateman, who argues, with reference to prostitution, that 'subordination is a *political* problem not a matter of morality, although moral questions are involved' (1988: 205). The debaters here treat adult–child sex as a problem of rights, but the argument is made on the grounds that there is an imposition of morality based on an unjustifiable division between adult and child sexuality. My point is that although these moral questions are involved, there are wider political questions; there are questions about power which the debaters gloss over, questions concerning age (generation), but also concerning gender.

To desire someone younger than oneself, with less access to power than oneself, is certainly not an abnormal desire. It is the predominant construction of masculine desire in the contemporary form of heterosexuality. If, therefore, one wishes to question the division between adult and child sexuality, one must also stress both the 'normality' of paedophilia and its gendered aspect. The debate draws attention to the fact that the law is involved in a demarcation of the boundaries of normal sexuality (i.e. even adult heterosexuality has boundaries concerning age/generation) and that involves a process of normalisation which maps out a space for the 'norm' by punishing the 'extremities'. But for all the arguments that speak up for children in the debate, it is not children who are imprisoned for such crimes, but the adults, or, rather, the *men* who commit them (on the whole). It is *they* who would be 'liberated' by the proposal. In this sense Foucault's proposal is not so much a radical proposal, as one that shores up the rights of the already most legally protected population – adult men – at least as far as age and gender are concerned.

Hocquenhem suggests: 'When we say that children are "consenting" in these cases, all we intend to say is this: in any case there was no violence, or organised manipulation in order to gain affective or erotic relations' (Foucault, 1988: 285). But how widely can we interpret the notion of 'organised manipulation'?

Whilst Foucault and the others succeed in raising the impossibility of answering the question 'how do you delineate a distinction between adult and child sexuality?', they move too quickly from 'you cannot' to 'you should not'. Whilst there is no watertight distinction between adult and child sexuality, and one can agree on some level with Foucault when he says 'an age barrier laid down by law does not have much sense' (1988: 284), it seems equally impossible to argue convincingly that there is *no* distinction, or that 'sexuality' is a constant across all ages. A constant *what*, we would have to ask? Is this another case of the 'forgotten whatness' of sexuality?

If one accepts that sexuality is constructed through contemporary discourse(s) that position children differently, then children *will* have a different understanding of their sexuality and their identities from adults. We are back to the 'bodies and pleasures'[3] problem. Is Foucault suggesting that children can and should be allowed to escape the strictures of their construction? Are they being constructed out of and away from a more fulfilling sexuality? This would not be a line of reasoning Foucault would wish to follow; it bears all the hallmarks of the perspective he made the target of his work. It seems almost as if Foucault and the others are suggesting that children have already 'escaped' such an understanding, or were never practising their sexuality in accordance with such an understanding. If this is their argument it seems that the debaters are asking for a legal acknowledgement of that 'escape'. However insoluble the theoretical questions that Foucault *et al.* ask, their proposal is highly unsatisfactory. At the very end of the discussion, Hocquenhem argues that 'we don't regard ourselves as legislators, but simply as a movement of opinion that demands the abolition of certain pieces of legislation' (in Foucault, 1988: 285). My suggestion is that the implications of what they propose, rather than signalling a victory for children's rights, or a radical cultural revision of the adult–child division, would be a victory for men in the realms of both sexuality and law.

Nevertheless, it would be misleading to pretend that this is an issue which feminism has completely resolved. If feminists support a law against adult–child relations it is because of an opposition to child sexual *abuse*. But feminist opposition to the proposal is framed in such a way that it involves making judgements about who can consent. Battles over age of consent laws in the history of feminism illustrate that feminist campaigns seeking to raise the age of consent to protect young women from sexual assault have dovetailed neatly with conservative morality movements (see, e.g., Jeffreys, 1985). The moral issues involved are not easy ones, and to pretend to have resolved them under the banner of feminism would be to deny their complexities. The important point in the debate is that it starts this process of questioning (for lawyers and for feminists), challenging the seemingly natural boundaries that law is involved in policing. For the time being, however, one might wish this questioning to stay at the level of academic questions rather than policy.

LOCATING SEX: ON RAPE

Introducing the issue of rape into a seminar on repression in 1977, Foucault (1988) presents a dilemma for comment. Although he believed as a matter of principle that 'in no circumstances should sexuality be subject to any kind of legislation whatever', rape is one area which 'for me present[s] a problem' (1988: 200). He goes on to argue:

One can always produce the theoretical discourse that

amounts to saying: in any case, sexuality can in no circumstances be the object of punishment. And when one punishes rape one should be punishing physical violence and nothing but that. And to say that it is nothing more than an act of aggression: that there is no difference, in principle, between sticking one's fist into someone's face or one's penis into their sex.

(1988: 200)

In effect, Foucault is arguing for a 'desexualisation' of rape,[4] a term he used himself in a slightly different context. In an interview Foucault once argued that the Women's Liberation Movement was a movement of 'desexualisation' because women were demanding that their lives no longer be addressed in terms of their sex, but that their situation be addresssed in terms of power inequalities since this is what 'the woman question' is really about:

The real strength of the women's movement is not that of having laid claim to the specificity of their sexuality and the rights pertaining to it, but that they have actually departed from the discourse conducted within the apparatuses of sexuality ... a veritable *desexualisation*, a displacement effected in relation to the sexual centring of the problem.

(1980a: 219)

In the seminar Foucault seems to suggest that his dilemma would be solved if rape were treated as an assault of violence and not as a sexual crime. But what is the source of his dilemma? Why should he wish to 'desexualise' rape? These questions are answered by placing Foucault's comments within the context of his arguments in *THS*. Although in the seminar Foucault presents his dilemma in terms of not wishing to legislate against sexuality, it becomes clear in the ensuing discussion that what he objects to is the construction of some part or parts of the body as 'sex' and as therefore special and in a sense more important than other parts of the body.

Foucault: The answer from both of you [the two women present] ... was very clear when I said: [rape] may be treated as an act of violence, possibly more serious, but of the same type, as that of punching someone in the face. Your answer was

161

immediately: No – its quite different. It's not just a punch in the face, but more serious.

Marine Zecca:[5] Of course!

Foucault: Then there are problems, because what we're saying amounts to this: sexuality as such, in the body, has a preponderant place, the sexual organ isn't like a hand, hair or a nose. It therefore has to be protected, surrounded, invested in any case with legislation that isn't pertaining to the rest of the body.

(Foucault, 1988: 201–2)

In this passage, Foucault provides a summary of the argument he understands his companions in the seminar to hold. He is asking them: what makes the genitalia so special? Why are they any different from another part of the body? Through their way of talking about sex, he is suggesting, sex is construed as located at certain parts of the body and, furthermore, as a special or privileged part of the body. It is with this way of talking and the legislation that perpetuates this way of talking that Foucault seems to be uncomfortable. Why?

It seems that Foucault sees this notion of sex as located in precise parts of the body as linked with the power/knowledge networks of the deployment of sexuality. Foucault had recently argued that power produces our understanding of the body, that the body is 'the inscribed surface of events' (1977: 148). Further, he had argued that the deployment of sexuality has elaborated the idea that 'there exists something other than bodies, organs, somatic localisations, functions, anatomo-physiological systems, sensations and pleasures; something else and something more, with intrinsic properties and laws of its own: "sex" ' (1981: 152–3). The argument in the debate on rape echoes this insofar as Foucault seems to be arguing that the discourses of the deployment of sexuality 'anchor' the concept of sexuality in the body by giving it a special place there.

As a resistance to the deployment of sexuality, then, Foucault seems to argue, we should refuse to see the sex of our bodies, i.e. the genitals, as anything more than or different from another part of the body, such as the fist or mouth. To treat rape as a sexual crime separates it out from other crimes of violence and colludes with the deployment of sexuality. It is from this perspective that Foucault is suggesting that rape should not be treated differently from a physical assault. To refuse to do so might undermine the power mechanisms around sexuality by exposing it as a free-floating construction. Rape, *insofar as its specificity rests upon a notion of the genitalia as different from and more important than other parts of the body,* as following different laws and requiring different treatment, is about the operations of power/knowledge and its ordering of the body. Refusing to take part in a legal discourse that is complicit with such an ordering is, from Foucault's perspective, a challenge to common sense understandings on which the deployment of sexuality relies.[6] If one pursues Foucault further by asking 'but why would one wish to challenge the deployment of sexuality like this?', Nancy Fraser's (1981; 1985) question of him, it seems that the answer would be that since sex has been set up as the key to our inner selves and the very truth of the individual, the desexualisation of rape would undermine the meaning of rape as such a grand transgression. It is this sense of an intimate attack upon the self that arguably makes rape so upsetting (Woodhull, 1988: 170).

The question that Foucault poses for feminist thought here touches upon a debate which has taken place within feminist circles and which has been formulated as either 'is rape about sex or power?' or 'is rape about sex or violence?'

One could argue that feminist thought has itself demanded a desexualisation of rape. Feminist work in the 1970s tended to argue that rape was an act of violence and was not about sex (Russell, 1975; Brownmiller, 1975; Griffin, 1982). Griffin argued: 'rape is an act of aggression in which the victim is denied her self-determination. *It is an act of violence* which, if not actually followed by beatings and murder, nevertheless always carries with it the threat of death' (1982: 57, emphasis added). As noted by De Lauretis (1987: 36), these analyses could therefore be regarded as employing a 'desexualisation' strategy similar to Foucault's. But is this position really the same as Foucault's?

The feminist position in the 1970s can be understood as a reaction against the ways in which rape was typically viewed (in court as well as by public opinion) as the result of a pent-up male sexual need. For example, Melani and Fodaski argued that 'rape is fundamentally an aggressive rather than a sexual act ... its motivation and dynamics arise out of hostility rather than sexual need' (1974: 82). Russell, too, argued that from the experiences recounted to her by survivors of rape, it seemed 'some rapists are not motivated by a sexual urge; the assertion of power over a woman seems more important' (1975: 260). Feminists argued that the fact that most rapes seem to be planned, to greater or lesser extent (Amir, 1971), undermined the notion that rape was the consequence of the man's overwhelming sexual need (Wilson, 1983: 65).

The pioneering feminist work of this period began, furthermore, to theorise rape as a political act. The New York Radical Feminists introduced their collection of conference papers thus:

> Through the technique of consciousness-raising, [we] discovered that rape is not a personal misfortune but an experience shared by all women in one form or another. When more than two people have suffered the same oppression the problem is no longer personal but political – and rape is a political matter.
>
> (Connell and Wilson, 1974: 1)

At around the same time, Brownmiller argued that rape was a mechanism by which men maintained their power over women. The fact that only a sub-set of men actually do rape women does not stop rape benefiting all men because all women are kept in fear: it is a process of intimidation that keeps all women wary of all men. Thus rape has a political function which is the maintenance of power of men over women.

If this early work employs a 'desexualisation' strategy to the extent that it argues that rape is not about sex, it might appear to be in agreement with Foucault's suggestion. Indeed, Canadian legal reform responded to feminist analyses by making rape a question of physical assault. In the place of the crime of rape they formulated a graduated scheme distinguishing sexual assaults purely in terms of the level of violence involved, and with no distinction between penetration and other sexual acts (Temkin, 1986: 34–5).

However, it is clear that this early feminist work on rape argued that rape is not about sex for reasons other than those put forward by Foucault. Whereas Foucault argues that rape is not about sex in order to *escape* power's operations which are surrounding and 'inscribing' the body, the feminist work argued that rape was not about sex in order to reveal and highlight the power relations and politics that are involved in rape and that had been ignored by legal and media discourse on rape. They argued that rape is not about sex but is *instead* about power. Foucault's argument is based upon the notion that by punishing only the violence of rape, by effectively collapsing the crime of rape into the crime of assault, one avoids those power deployments which would have one regard rape as sexual. The feminist argument, on the other hand, was that rape should be analytically divorced from sex in order to show how the act of rape is motivated not by sexual desire but by power and, furthermore, occupies a privileged position in its connection with the operations and maintenance of power. Clearly, there are different analyses behind what may at first glance appear the same 'desexualisation' strategy.

Moreover, there was always an ambivalence in the feminist 'not sex, power' or 'violence not sex' claims, as evident in Peterson's statement: 'rape is first and foremost a crime of violence against the body and only secondarily (*although importantly*) a sex crime' (1977: 364; emphasis added). This ambivalence left room for manouevre, and the feminist position has shifted 'back' again. Later feminist texts have argued that rape is about sex. One can approach this debate through a discussion of the response to Foucault.

Monique Plaza (1980) has confronted Foucault on his comments on rape.[7] Plaza argues that rape *is* about sex, and cannot be treated as if it were the same as a punch in the face. Rape is commonly regarded as sexual in the sense that it involves the genitals, but Plaza argues that this is not what leads her to argue, *contra* Foucault, that rape is a sexual crime which should be regarded as such. Rape does not have to involve the genitals, she contends, since the introduction of a bottle held by a man into the anus of a woman would also be rape. Her argument is not that more areas of the body need to be regarded as sexual, but that attention needs to be directed away from parts of the body and toward the actors involved. It is 'social sexing' which makes rape sexual, she argues, meaning that it opposes men and women, members of the two sexes. Thus: 'rape is an oppressive practice employed by a (social) man against a (social) woman' (1980: 31).

The parenthetical term 'social' is used by Plaza to convey her belief that although a man can also be raped, in the process he is placed in the position of a woman. That is, 'the anus of a man can be placed in the position of "the sex" or, furthermore, a (biological) man can be put in the place of the "body of women" and can be appropriated as such' (1980: 31). Thus she argues that when a man is raped, he is constituted as feminine by that act. Her argument is that one has therefore to discuss rape in terms of gender. It is *social* sex, not biological sex, that rape is 'about'.

Plaza suggests that Foucault has overlooked his own argument in *THS* where he speaks of the three ways in which sex has been defined

> [A]s that which belongs in common to both men and women; as that which belongs *par excellence* to men, and hence is lacking in women; but at the same time as that which by itself constitutes woman's body, ordering it in terms of the functions of reproduction.
>
> (1981: 153)

If men rape women, argues Plaza, it is precisely because they are women in the social sense, because they are 'the sex'. She suggests:

> Men rape women insofar as they belong to a class of men who have appropriated the bodies of women. They rape what they have learnt to consider their property ... the class of women (which ... can also contain biological men).
>
> (1980: 32)

Plaza also justifies her rejection of Foucault's arguments using a different line of attack. She contends that, in practical terms, taking rape out of its present place in law, as Foucault advocates, would mean permitting rape; she argues her point by suggesting that responses to a physical assault and to rape are very different. Punching someone in the face is generally conceived as a criminal assault, and one would generally expect sympathetic treatment if one wished to report the offender to the police. On the other hand, because placing the penis in the vagina is not an action generally considered as an assault, but is defined as heterosexual intercourse, reporting rape to the authorities sets in motion a series of questions that runs 'but you have no lesions, where is the sperm? you did not consent? where are your witnesses?' (1980: 32). Rape, because of its (debatable) imitation of a legal behaviour, would just not be dealt with in the same way as a physical assault. Furthermore, Foucault's suggestion would exacerbate an existing problem because rape is already treated as a physical assault to the extent that it is to evidence of violence that the authorities look in order to distinguish rape from consensual heterosexual intercourse.

Plaza argues that women are the hardest hit by the 'machinery' of the deployment of sexuality described by Foucault, and that they cannot afford to jump into the realm of the ideal and pretend that, here and now, sex (the genitals) is the same as other parts of the body. Thus Plaza would agree with the position that Foucault summarises disapprovingly: '[Sex] must ... be protected, surrounded, at any rate, provided with legislation which does not apply to the rest of the body' (1988: 202).

Whether or not it is possible to evaluate the impact and prove that women are the hardest hit by the deployment of sexuality (it seems unlikely that such a quantification makes much sense), it is clear that the most effective weapon that Plaza has against Foucault is in the illustration that, in practice and at present, the implementation of his ideas would work to the detriment of the woman raped (Stern, 1980). Importantly, Plaza states that she has no quarrel with the ideas in themselves. In fact, she argues that they are in part 'abstractly (idealistically) correct' (1980: 28). This, she suggests, is what makes them all the more pernicious. Her critique stages a politicisation of Foucault's remarks, looking at the implications from the raped women's point of view, and this leads her to suggest, in reference to *The Archaeology of Knowledge* (1972), that Foucault has not considered the 'enuciative mode' of his own discourse, a term he defined as the place from which the author of a discourse speaks, giving coherence to what s/he says.

Through a different argument, Catherine MacKinnon (1982; 1987; 1989) also (re)introduces the term 'sex' into feminist debates on rape. She argues that the umbrella term 'violence against women' fails to criticise sex and the ways in which women have been oppressed through sex. Whilst MacKinnon's position is indicative of a general shift in feminist approaches to violence against women (Edwards, 1987), the issue of desexualisation does not seem to be simply a case of evolving feminist opinion. There are not just two positions here – the early and the later feminist position, the first in agreement with Foucault and the later in disagreement – but several. But the debate is in danger of collapsing both because there are different meanings accorded to the term 'sex' such that those who are arguing that rape is about sex can actually hold quite different perspectives (as can those who argue that it is not), and because the question has been set up as if there were only the possibility that rape is *either* about sex *or* about power *or* about violence, whereas most arguments involve all three terms in some form or another.

First, therefore, one has to address the different meanings being attributed to the term 'sex'. Both Plaza and MacKinnon argue that sex should be brought into the feminist discussions, but they do so *without* being in agreement with the sort of 'rape is about sex' position that the earlier feminist position was directed against. The 'sex' that they bring back in is not the same 'sex' that was thrown out by earlier feminists; nor is it the same 'sex' that Foucault wishes to challenge. There are in fact at least three ways in which the term 'sex' is used in this whole debate:

1 *It is used to refer to the anatomy.* Foucault's point is that sex has been constructed as located at discrete areas of the body. To 'take sex out of rape', for him, means to deprivilege the genitals. This meaning of sex is not absent from feminist work, for feminists have also 'decentred' the genitals, arguing that other forms of assault can be just as serious.

2 *It is used to refer to sexuality/sexual desire.* When early feminist work argued that rape is not about sex but about power or violence, they were often arguing that sexual desire was not the motivation behind rape (Melani and Fodaski, 1974; Russell, 1975). There was also the argument that rape certainly did not feel like sex to the woman. These arguments employ the term 'sex' to mean sexual desire or sexuality. Later feminist work has argued that, on the contrary, sexual desire is involved. Barry argues that 'in committing a crime against women, sexual satisfaction, usually in the form of orgasm, is one of the intended outcomes of sexual violence for the aggressor' (1985: 164). Other feminist work has argued that the social construction of masculine sexuality must form the backdrop to a feminist analysis of rape. Thus MacKinnon argues that violence and power are entwined in the male sexual role which 'centres on aggressive intrusion on those with less power. Such acts of domination are experienced as sexually arousing, as sex itself' (1989: 127). Invoking Foucault's comments, she states 'a feminist analysis would suggest that assault by a man's fist is not so different from

assault by a penis not because both are violent but because both are sexual' (1989: 178). Because force is experienced as sexually exciting, MacKinnon argues that force is 'the desire dynamic, not just a response to the desired object when desire's expression is frustrated' (1989: 186).

In this sense, therefore, sex means sexuality or sexual desire, and rape is 'about sex' because the man's sexuality is an important part of the picture. Using the same sense, but taking a different line of approach, Dumaresq (1981) has argued that rape is about sex because it is the site at which discourses converge to create a specific sexuality of 'the rape victim'. The media and judicial discourses on rape, she suggests, centre on the sexual intent/desire of the woman, inquiring into her dress, behaviour and sexual history, thereby discursively constructing a sexuality of the 'true' rape victim. In the rape trial, Dumaresq suggests that men's and women's sexualities are constructed within a specific set of discursive practices that do not operate elsewhere. For this reason she suggests rape must be analysed as sexual, for to do otherwise would be to miss the ways in which rape is linked with constructions of the specific sexuality of the rape victim and the man who is likely to have raped.

The sex-as-sexuality use of the term 'sex' has been an important one in the 'desexualisation' debate, one that traverses several different positions.

3   *The third usage of the term 'sex' refers to gender.* Plaza's argument is that rape is sexual because it opposes men and women, it is 'about' the ways in which masculine will treat feminine within present power relations. Further, Plaza suggests that rape is about gendered 'positionalities' since a man can take the position of a woman in rape. Rape is about sex, therefore, because it is 'about' gender relations. Divorced from the referent of genitalia, sex becomes gender and gender becomes behaviour; rape is about sex because it is about the ways in which masculine people (who tend to have the genitalia that is recognised as male) are taught to treat women (who, similarly, tend to have the genitalia that is recognised as female).

This is a different usage of the term from the 'sex' that Foucault argues rape should no longer be about, from the 'sex' that early feminists argued rape is not about *and* from the 'sex' that MacKinnon argues rape is about.

These different usages of the term 'sex' have served to confuse this whole debate. The same answer to the question 'is rape about sex?' can in fact disguise widely divergent perspectives. Moreover, opposing answers can disguise a similar position.

The debate runs deeper into conceptual muddles because whilst it has been set up as if it involved one term, i.e. whether rape is (or should be theorised as) about sex or not, or as if it involved two, i.e. 'is rape about sex or violence?', there are in fact *three* terms at stake: sex, power and violence. It is the way in which the contributors map their perspectives onto this triangle of terms that differentiates them. Foucault argues that to escape power rape should be desexualised and treated as violent assault. How does this compare with the feminist positions?

Early feminist work on rape argued that rape was not about sex in order to challenge the belittling of rape as an encounter comparable with one of mutual desire; violence was a term used to move the argument away from discussions of sex and onto discussions of assault. Power is seen as a relevant concept in these early feminist texts for three different reasons. First, because a power structure is held to exist between groups such as men and women, with rape a tool used to maintain this structure (Brownmiller; 1975; Griffin, 1982). Secondly, the desire to feel powerful is held to form at least part of a man's motivation to rape; he rapes to experience the power of making another human being do as he wishes against her will (Russell, 1975). Thirdly, it is theorised as the context in which rape takes place. That is, the fact that a man can rape a woman is an illustration and expression of the fact that he has power over her. This is perhaps at its most clear when the man is known to the woman or related to her so that even before the rape it is understood that she will or should obey his orders.

For these early feminist positions, therefore, as for Foucault, 'violence' is a discursive solution, a term used to take emphasis away from the term 'sex'. But the feminist position is not the same as Foucault's. In stressing the violence of rape, feminists were stressing the violation of the person (Peterson, 1977). This invokes the notion that Foucault was trying to subvert, i.e. that rape attacks the self. The use of the term power in the feminist accounts, moreover, depicts power's operations differently from Foucault.

Plaza's contribution illustrates the limitations of the term 'violence' as a discursive solution by suggesting that it cannot convey the full feminist position and risks being misread as a denial of the most basic feminist argument on the issue: that rape is about the social relations between men and women. Plaza seems to want to give up the term violence in order to analyse rape in terms of power relations between the genders. The work of Dumaresq is much closer to Foucault because she is drawing upon his work in her discussion of the discursive construction of the rape victim. It therefore uses the notion of power in a much more Foucauldian way. Ironically, however, she would be put on the opposite side of the fence from Foucault if the division were around the question 'is rape about sex?' or, more accurately, 'should we analyse rape as about sex?'

MacKinnon would be difficult to place on one or other side of such a division for although she writes 'against' those who would see rape as simply violence, her argument that the relations between power, sex and violence are entwined at the site of 'normal' male sexuality refuses the 'sex or violence' question. In her analysis, all three terms are relevant and imply each other. Thus she states: 'to the extent that coercion has become integral to male sexuality, rape may even be sexual to the degree that, and because, it is violent' (1989: 173). MacKinnon's usage of the triangle of terms means that in effect she refuses to take sides in the way the debate has been set up.

QUESTIONS WITHOUT ANSWERS

A central problem that arises in both these debates is how difference is discursively created. In the first debate the difference between adult sexuality and child sexuality is interrogated, and in the second the difference between the 'sexual' and other parts of the body. In turn, the second debate raises the question of the difference between men and women. Rosi Braidotti has argued that Foucault bypasses the challenge that psychoanalysis has addressed, that is, that the subject is not universal but sexed, gender specific. For him it is 'as if the notion of human being ... is neutralised when it comes to sexual difference' (Braidotti, 1991: 95). Whilst Foucault's retort would be that his task is to pose questions about how we discursively create differences within and between bodies, it is undeniable that his position in these two debates leaves an uncomfortable question mark over the issue of difference. By criticising the continued articulation of difference within legal discourse, Foucault implies that a sameness would be preferable. It is not an argument about the instrinsic qualities of bodies since he nowhere suggests that all bodies and all sexual experiences are the same. Rather, it is a *legal* sameness that Foucault seems to advocate. His question is why, how and with what consequences have we understood these parts of the body and these 'sexualities' as different?

When it comes to questions of legislation, however, of bringing about change in legal discourse, the problem with the 'only asking' position is forced to centre-stage. Foucault is actually laying his cards on the table, aligning himself with a 'movement of opinion', even if he reserves the right to alter them in the next moment. In the first debate discussed in this chapter, the 'natural' boundary that Foucault *et al.* question is the adult/child distinction in terms of sexuality; in the second it is the boundaries within the body between sexual and non-sexual areas. Foucault's questions draw attention to the ways in which stubborn discursive categorisation has consequences both within and beyond the legal sphere. In the move from descriptive to prescriptive, however, Foucault appears to envisage an escape from these particular discursive categories. In proposing an alternative way of speaking, a discourse of non-differentiation, Foucault is at his most idealistic, arguing that his suggestions would improve the legal and wider social understanding of adult–child relations and rape. His questions are certainly striking and draw attention to the creation of discursive categories and processes of power/ knowlege. He forces a consideration of questions that have been avoided: Why is the sexed body always a given in discussions of rape? Why is the possibility of a child consenting defined out of discussions of adult–child sex? It is true that these questions are central but have not really been debated in any depth in feminist discussions.

It is in the explication of his solutions that Foucault's position becomes so frustrating. The frustration arises because the two concepts Foucault appears to address – 'consent' and 'sex' – become curiously decontextualised as he posits strategies for legal reform. The strategies are presented as 'escapes' from discursive constructions but without discussion of the new formulations that are thereby instituted. These new formulations, I have argued, may appear remarkably familiar to feminist onlookers. As Naomi Schor has remarked, whilst Foucault may be interested in 'limit-cases of difference' and he may dream of getting beyond constructed differences, we have 'to construct a post-deconstructionist society that will not simply reduplicate our own' (1987: 110).

7

CONCLUSION

What if the 'object' started to speak?

(Irigaray, 1985: 135)

Incest is an issue on which the 'object' *has* started to speak, and this book has been about the ways in which we can think about that speech. Feminism has provided a discursive space enabling survivors of incest to speak and to be heard, and the setting up of help lines and women's centres has provided a much needed channel of communication. (Re)emerging through these efforts, the 'subjugated knowledges' of incest survivors have formed the foundations of the feminist understanding of incest. From these accounts of pain, courage and resistance, issues familiar from previous feminist discussions of sexual violence have arisen, and, as a consequence, the feminist analyses have placed incest within a generalised theory of patriarchal power and sexual violence, analysing it more or less according to a model of rape. Part of the task of the feminist analyses has been to highlight 'myths' of incest, to offer an alternative account of incest, as well as to generate statistics on the prevalence and forms of sexual abuse. In short, something we might call a 'feminist knowledge' has appeared and, simultaneously, the object of that knowledge: 'incestuous abuse'.[1]

This knowledge has simultaneously grown out of and provided a basis for the provision of feminist support to women survivors of incest. Since feminism is not just about organising support, however, but incorporates social critique, feminists have engaged in challenging other forms of knowledge around the issue of incest. That is, feminist thought has entered into discursive battles around the meaning of 'incest'. Some of these battles resemble those undertaken with respect to other forms of sexual violence. For example, attacking the casting of women and girls into a whore/madonna dichotomy has been a common task. On the other hand, some are peculiar to incest, mainly because of the varied discourses which converge around it. Casting incest as an issue of sexual violence has to a certain extent meant that feminist analyses have not detailed the challenge their work represents to these other ways of speaking about incest. Whilst the reasons for approaching incest in this way are good ones, feminism has effectively defined certain specific concepts such as the incest taboo as outside its remit and defined itself out of the sociological debates that have taken place around incest. In the preceding pages I have returned the feminist analyses to the sociological questions surrounding the incest prohibition and to socio-legal questions around the criminalisation of incest.

Although feminists may not have directly addressed the question of how their work on incest as sexual violence threatens previous sociological preoccupations, insofar as feminist understanding of incest is located in the practices of social life and not just within academic debate nor within the covers of books, there have been several discursive battles in which feminist understandings of incest have met sociological and other understandings. Measuring the success of feminist knowledge in these discursive battles is a precarious business. Within sociology, it would seem that feminism has won a discursive battle in the sense that discussions of incest are expected to address questions of sexual violence and not the origin or function of the incest prohibition. Outside the academy, too, the issue of child sexual abuse within the family is now taken seriously within media, social work and legal discussions in a way that it has not been in previous eras. It is not too controversial to suggest that feminism has been the most prominent movement in the current drive to put incest on the agenda. Once incest moves out of feminist discourse and practices and into these other arenas, however, it is difficult to know how 'feminist' these moves remain. Where feminist arguments reinforce arguments made within child protection, welfarist and charity discourses, they have been part of a powerful collective force. This seems to be the case both in the criminalisation of incest, as I have discussed, and in the recent moves to make court procedures less intimidating for children. However, feminist knowledge has a specificity that is in danger of being lost if it is conflated with these discourses. The feminist becomes seen as just another 'welfarist' voice and another version of a 'save the children' position. Set up in this way, moreover, it is positioned as an incomplete analysis, focusing, as it predominantly has done, on only the girl survivors. Attempts to deny the necessity of a feminist perspective frequently base their claims on the evidence of the sexual abuse of boy children.[2] The argument is that if all children are vulnerable to abuse, this is not a feminist issue. This misses the point that the feminist position is not just about highlighting the sexual damage suffered by girls and women but simultaneously forms a fundamental critique of the family, of the construction of gendered sexualities, of the 'normality' of incestuous abuse. All this pertains to the abuse of both girls and boys. The specific contribution of the feminist perspective is that it locates the problem of incest within the normal practices of sexuality, of power and of practices of 'not-hearing'. Its task has been to show the gendered and generational quality of these practices.

When one starts to question how the feminist position conflicts, supports and is conflated with other ways of speaking about incest, one places feminist work within the terrain which Foucault made his object of study. With his argument that talk about sex, including talk about sexual violence, is not liberatory as advertised but indicates the operations of the power/knowledge networks of the deployment of sexuality, Foucault implicitly casts the feminist work within his scenario, as sharing archaic understandings of power, freedom and discourse, understandings that not only misrepresent but actually contribute to the present bio-political system.

For the most part, the feminist response to the challenge of Foucault's work has taken place at a general theoretical level, and has consisted largely of attempts to enclose one body of work within the other. That is, on the one hand some feminists have suggested that feminists can regard Foucault as another male theorist and can file him alongside previous male thinkers. Having filed Foucault, the choice is then either to ignore him, or to use his work, to pick up and mould his concepts and arguments to see whether they illuminate a point or situation. On the other hand, some have treated feminism as inescapably within the Foucauldian filing cabinet, and have argued that feminism must therefore proceed by negotiating that position.

With this latter move, feminism is forced to reflect upon its status as a knowledge, its relationship with other discourses and to consider lines of resistance within those that uphold the injustices feminism seeks to challenge. Simultaneously feminism has to be resigned to the understanding that it contains all the contradictions and power/knowledge links that other ways of speaking contain. One cannot maintain this notion of filing cabinets for long simply because neither feminism nor the work of Foucault could be contained within an enclosed space in the way that metaphor suggests. It is not only that Foucault's work has influenced what 'feminism' contains,[3] nor that they have both necessarily been influenced by similar ways of speaking (Marxism, for example), but that they are ways of understanding the social world that are reproduced and circulate in the same space. To try to decide which is the 'bigger', which can contain and explain the other, seems to be a pointless exercise that relies on some impossible conception of the 'size' of each. Nevertheless, the image enables one to consider the evaluative procedures that are put into operation: sometimes Foucault is set up as explaining feminism, sometimes feminism is the testing ground for Foucault. There is clearly a case for exploring both directions. In this book neither Foucault nor feminism has been set up as the acid test of the other, for although both ask pertinent questions about real issues, neither has all the answers. Rather than attempting to reach a satisfactory merger between the two on this general level, this book has explored how the two converge and conflict on specific questions.

By focusing on the one topic, that of incest, this book has attempted to break away from the generality of the 'Foucault and feminism' debate and to focus on details such as the way feminist analyses have conveyed the operations of power in incestuous abuse, the detail of Foucault's arguments about the convergence of two systems around incest, the details of the criminalisation of incest. In doing so it has utilised both the approaches to Foucault, using his work as a pool of ideas which feminism can borrow and use in the exploration of territories of interest to feminism, and exploring the implications of regarding feminist work on incest as 'within' the Foucauldian landscape.

The encounter with Foucault on the specific example of incest has meant a rethinking of the feminist approach to power, sexuality and 'myths'. Much of this rethinking has not entailed change in the basic feminist approach to incest as a problem of sexual violence, but has simply used Foucault as a site at which to clarify the feminist position. The striking image of panoptical power has been used in feminist work on femininity, and seems particularly pertinent in incestuous abuse where looking and sexual pleasure are closely linked, and where power mechanisms control the movement of the abused, who are both objectified and subjectified as 'docile' bodies. Resisting that objectification has meant working against these forms of intrafamilial power. There are also places where the feminist work raises questions about Foucault's position. For example, juridico-discursive power does seem to be an appropriate model to use in an analysis of the ways in which Fathers exercise power in the household, even where disciplinary techniques can also be discerned, but Foucault does not really make clear what his response would be to such a discussion, seeming at times uncertain about whether juridico-discursive power has disappeared, whether it never trully existed (and was just an image projected by those whose power actually operated in different ways) or is still alive and kicking but somewhat subdued by more recent techniques of bio-power.

The concurrence of feminist and Foucauldian arguments on sexuality are revealed in the critique that both pursue of the normal/pervert distinction, and in a general position that sexual practices are discursively informed. Foucault's work provides an opportunity to work through the feminist stance, and to consider how the 'myths' form networks of talk and practice around and about 'incest'. Whatever one might think of the place of emancipatory politics in Foucault's thesis, his depiction of power/ knowledge strategies strengthens the feminist approach to incest by shining a light on how these knowledges create personages that, held up as perverse and abnormal, can protect the 'normality' of other practices: normal masculine sexuality, the normal protective head of the household, the normal caring mother, the normal functioning family, and so on. As feminist work illustrates, the normal is as much constructed, as 'mythical', as the abnormal. When seen as a sexual abuse, incest is a subject that threatens to reveal the mechanisms at work in maintaining the 'traditional' discourses around sexuality, children and the family.

However, as I have suggested, the feminist approach is not the only way in which incest is 'put into discourse'. One of the central arguments of this book is that incest is not a unitary phenomenon. The suggestion here is not that incest takes many forms, but that incest is a constructed category, not an act, and that construction can take many forms. Echoing the arguments stemming from labelling theory, one might say what makes an act incestuous is how we label it. What is incest . . . which relations, what movements, with what sentiment? Bringing a Foucauldian perspective to bear on this point, one begins to ponder the power/knowledge networks that surround and deploy the category 'incest'. For feminism incest is a problem of sexual violence, for others it is a problem of the genetic consequences of inbreeding, for others it is about housing, for others child protection is the rallying cry, and so on. Although from a Foucauldian angle, therefore, the feminist analyses are viewed as one way of speaking about incest amongst many, this is not a matter of dissolving feminist politics by accepting all ways of speaking as equally correct. Rather, it is a question of recognising that feminism has problematised incest in a particular way but is forced to enter into a discursive space where several different understandings of what incest is about are reproduced. Instead of asking what makes one way of understanding incest better than another, the Foucauldian task is to study the relations between these ways of understanding incest, to treat the exercise as a study of the problematisation of incest.

Hacking has argued that there are 'few fundamental concepts that we can watch being made and moulded before our eyes' (1991: 286) but that child abuse is such a concept, one which has been medicalised as an abnormal practice in the twentieth century. Incest has changed its meaning as it has been appended to the notion of child abuse, Hacking suggests, so that what counts as incest, and what counts as abuse, is 'tied to other current practices and sensibilities' (1991: 277). In exposing and talking about the issue of incest, feminists necessarily enter the domain of talk that defines and redefines social problems. The task, then, is to consider how feminist knowledge operates there. I have argued that one can both continue to operate within the feminist parameters of meaning and values and also understand one's position as historically specific and subject to change. Foucault's warning that one may be involved in the reproduction of modes of power and categories of normal/abnormal does not give clues as to how one knows when and how one is involved in those networks. Sawicki notes that Foucault's suggestion that 'our discourses can extend relations of domination at the same time that they are critical of them' provides not an alternative theory but 'a way of looking at our theories of self and society and a method of re-evaluating them' (1991: 10–11). There is no contradiction between using Foucault and refusing to take him as the standard of truth; if feminist work on incest is located as a discourse on sex about which Foucault was writing, as I believe it must be, that is not the same as saying that everything else he said about that condition is to be accepted without question. One way of 'looking at' those theories is to attempt to monitor them as they are articulated; another is to mount an investigation into how they operate or have operated.

In the process of criminalisation various ways of speaking about incest came together. I have discussed the criminalisation of incest in order to interrogate the meeting of these different and oftentimes conflicting understandings of what incest is 'about'. How were these ways of speaking articulated in the process of constructing the legal object 'incest'? Analysis of the parliamentary debates illustrates the sense in which there are many contrasting 'incests' being placed on the table for consideration. There were the traditional objections to incest, assertions that repeatedly place incest on the side of the 'forbidden', but alongside these assertions are the arguments of bio-political knowledges that present incest as something whose form is to be studied and detailed and whose wrong is measurable. The processes involve a mapping out of a specific place for incest as a crime. Its wrong is equivalent not to that of rape, nor to that of child abuse, but to something else, something that requires separate legislation: hence the law of incest. The messiness of the discursive battle is denied by the criminalisation of incest through a simple statement of prohibition, most clearly in the English legislation, in which 'incest' is placed clearly on the side of the forbidden as if tradition or reactionary morality were all that had informed it.

The Scottish legislation betrays traces of the impact of child-centred, protectionist discourses that coincide at certain points with the feminist position, since it includes as incest intercourse between a parent and adopted child and as 'related' offences intercourse between a step-child and step-parent and sexual abuse by unrelated members of the household, specifying age limits for the child. These additions indicate the criminal-isation has had a slightly more messy passage than would be the case if the legislation were merely the reproduction of a 'thou shalt not commit incest' command.

Carol Smart has argued that an analysis of how the law operates in the maintenance or otherwise of gender relations needs to be attuned to the contradictions within law and legal practice at every level. With reference to earlier feminist analyses of law,[4] she argues that

> to conceptualise the law as a repressive tool of a patriarchal state is an oversimplification of the role of law in sustaining the social order. I do not see the law simply as a conservative force. . . . On the contrary, law itself is seen as multifaceted system of regulation, containing its own contradictions, and most importantly, capable of change and positive influence rather than just negative restraint.
>
> (1984: 221)

Smart suggests the law is not a tool of some greater power such as 'patriarchy', and proposes that law be considered in its specificity rather than its generality in order to see in what sense the law 'makes a claim to truth . . . [which] is indivisible from the exercise of power' (1989: 11).[5]

Legislation appears simply to respond, perhaps slowly, perhaps inadequately, to reality, and feminists frequently call upon law to respond to realities that it does not seem to recognise. However, once an issue is taken into the legal process, it is subject to a process of definition and redefinition that draws in various knowledges, and is pushed and pulled onto various agendas. It may well be the case that feminist agitation, joining with charitable and/or welfarist interest, put incest onto the legal agenda, both in the early part of this century and more recently with the review of an ancient and archaic Scots law, but the debates studied here suggest that, in terms of shaping the legal object, feminism is a relatively weak voice when placed in contention with some powerful scientific, psychological and moralistic knowledges. Nevertheless, a feminist understanding is articulated and the possibility of its articulation gives cause for optimism, indicating that feminist understandings can have some impact on the processes by which law defines its truths. Smart illustrates the way in which the construction of truth takes place in the courtroom, where the 'psy' professionals can be drawn into the process of legal decision-making, and this is a process affecting cases of incest as any other. My focus, however, has been on the formulation of statutory law where the legal object 'incest' is created out of the discursive battles; a discursive construction that has been created or 'moulded' through the conflicts and conflation of several different understandings. It is therefore a product, and not a response. The emerging legislation does not so much respond to a reality as define that reality through its decisions about what will constitute incest in law. Since legal discourse has a certain status, this understanding can in turn structure further discussions on the issue.

The contrast between the various bio-political knowledges and the simple authoritative statement of prohibition reflects the disjunction to which Foucault drew attention in his comments on incest. For although the approach to incest as an issue of problematisation is in danger of becoming a simple descriptive task, Foucault placed incest at a central theoretical position in terms of the general operations of bio-power in modern societies. As I have suggested, its centrality is due in turn to the role of the family in the dissemination of power/knowledge techniques of the deployment of sexuality. Incest is precisely the issue around which Foucault suggests the 'old', traditional ways of speaking about sex remain important as the newer bio-political ways of speaking encroach. The crime of incest appears to be a classic example of the old mode of power, but is in fact informed by these newer ways of speaking about sex. Thus this 'old' mode of speaking has been reinstituted in the midst of the period in which Foucauldians would expect to find power operating bio-politically; a 'traditional' prohibition kept alive via newer ways of speaking.

Foucault implies that the deployment of alliance 'reacted' to the deployment of sexuality, that insistence on the importance of an incest taboo has been a fearful reaction to the effects of the power/knowledge networks surrounding the family, discourses that by their attention to the sexuality of those within the household served to incite incest. The feminist analyses of incest have themselves adopted the argument that discourses incite sexual behaviour with reference to both acceptable sexual behaviour and abusive sexual behaviour, explaining incestuous abuse in terms of the intersection of accepted discourses, especially those of authority in the household and masculine sexuality. Foucault's argument, however, places feminist work on the same level as the discourses it criticises, regarding it as part of the discursive noise around the family and sex. The Foucauldian hypothesis turns the tables on feminist work in this way, suggesting that these efforts may not be as unproblematically progressive as their proponents would wish. There are of course contradictions in the position the feminist work occupies: it intends to be part of the movement that gets people talking about sexual abuse and intends that talk becomes incorporated into effective action. In doing so, it is frequently co-opted into what Foucauldians would label bio-political strategies, the 'policing of the family', constructing sexual problems and fuelling the escalating discourse on sex and the family. Although it joins other discourses on sexual practices and joins an attention to the household unit, however, the feminist work remains critical such that it also operates as a counter-discourse, in particular in the way it interrupts the discourse to question the normal/abnormal divisions central to the deployment of sexuality.

Part of the risk in Foucault's work, and one of the reasons that his work has sometimes received a frosty welcome, is in this questioning of the radicalism of radical movements. Foucault suggested that in academic work and in everyday life we should consistently question the obviousness of categories and pro-cedures that are deployed around us, and that one's own convictions and beliefs should not escape this questioning. In the debates on adult–child sex and rape, Foucault displayed his ability to pose questions around such taken-for-grantedness. I have suggested that his skill in this role points to certain issues that are taken for granted, both generally and within feminist debates. As individuals, we reproduce and reconstruct the discourses by which we live, and although feminism can be a means by which women and men construct their lives differently, it is not surprising that it can also perpetuate certain ways of talking. Addressing the questions of consent in relation to children, and of the differentiation of the sexed parts of the body from the rest, Foucault illuminates areas of debate that have received little attention within the feminist work on sexual violence. They are, moreover, areas that need to be addressed, because, for example, the movement toward letting children 'speak for themselves' in law has been welcomed by feminists, but we may soon be faced with ethico-political decisions around whether and how children's evidence should be treated differently from adults'. The meaning of consent has not been clarified in feminist debates on rape, and in debates on child sexual abuse it tends to disappear because it is subordinated to a rigid understanding of power hierarchies. Thus although Foucault's position can ultimately be dismissed as unsatisfactory, his comments do highlight this lack of feminist discussion around consent. With regard to the debate on rape, the conclusion is similar. That is, Foucault's arguments force a discussion around the status of the body in feminist work, and how that relates to ways of speaking about gender and sex. The current interest in the discursive production of the body, partly inspired by Foucault, may force this confrontation with feminist work on sexual violence.

However, as soon as Foucault takes the 'ethico-political' decision, a plan of action, he lines himself up with other movements of opinion and, in both cases, against a generalised feminist position. Foucault does not convince that now is the time to challenge the particular discursive differentiations he addresses. The image he presents does not appeal to the feminist reading the debates now, in the context of feminist activity on the issue of sexual violence, for in his radicalism one can see the shape of rather too familiar problems. The dissolution of the legal differentiations Foucault addresses would be, one suspects, a temporary victory for him and another hurdle for survivors of sexual violence.

There are feminists who have completely refused to give Foucault space, seeing his popularity as another example of hero worship within the male canon. Others have provided detailed critiques of Foucault's politics characterising his work as inherently conservative and dangerous. The worries are by now well rehearsed – that refusing to identify structures of power and domination will mean the loss of radical oriented politics, that questioning our fundamental terms of identity will mean losing the impetus behind political groupings, and so on. These arguments tend to rely to a greater or lesser extent upon a pragmatism of the form 'if we theorise like that, how can we do this?' The problem here is that the wish to remain 'political' has led not so much to a rebuttal of Foucault's theoretical arguments

184

as to a refusal of them in terms of feminism's political aims. In this study of Foucault and feminism I have focused on the crime of incest in order to explore their theoretical relationship on a concrete issue, looking at the resulting configurations seriously but sceptically. By throwing these ingredients together, uncomfortable questions and important dilemmas are raised, but the exploration as a whole has argued that there are also striking convergences and powerful shared lines of critique. The questioning of post-structuralism currently divides feminists, but the threatening figure of the post-structuralist theorist tends to be drawn at 'twice its natural size'.[6] Exploring the work of Foucault may have cast a different light on the feminist work on incest, but it has diminished neither its force nor, sadly, its continuing relevance.

APPENDIX I
The law of incest in Britain

ENGLISH LAW

Incest is criminalised by the Sexual Offences Act 1956 which incorporated the Punishment of Incest Act 1908.

Incest is committed by a man when he has sexual intercourse (defined as the penetration of the vagina by the penis) with a woman whom he knows to be his grand-daughter, daughter, sister or mother. 'Sister' includes half-sister. These relationships need not be traced through 'lawful wedlock'. (s10).

Incest is committed by a woman of the age of sixteen or over when she permits a man whom she knows to be her grandfather, father, brother or son to have sexual intercourse with her by her consent. 'Brother' includes half-brother. These relationships need not be traced through 'lawful wedlock'. (s11).

Relationships by adoption are not covered. However, if D has sexual intercourse with E whom he believes to be his sister, when she is in fact adopted, he will be guilty of attempt.

The mens *rea* of incest requires knowledge of the relationship (but not that the relationship is criminalised as incest).

When the girl is under thirteen (and the indictment specifically alleges this) the offence is punishable with life imprisonment and an attempt is punishable with seven years imprisonment. In all other cases the maximum sentences are seven years for the full offence and two years for attempt.

SCOTS LAW

Incest is criminalised by the Incest and Related Offences (Scotland) Act 1986.

Incest is committed by any man or woman who has sexual intercourse with any person who is related to her as specified in the table below, unless s/he: did not know s/he was so related; or, did not consent to sexual intercourse or to sexual intercourse with that person; or, was married to that person by a marriage entered into outside Scotland and recognised as valid by Scots law.

For males	For females
1. Relationships by consanguinity	
Mother	Father
Daughter	Son
Grandmother	Grandfather
Grand-daughter	Grandson
Sister	Brother
Aunt	Uncle
Niece	Nephew
Great grandmother	Great grandfather
Great grand-daughter	Great grandson
2. Relationships by adoption	
Adoptive mother or former adoptive mother	Adoptive father or former adoptive father
Adoptive daughter or former adoptive daughter	Adoptive son or former adoptive son

These relationships are criminal whether they are of the full blood or the half blood, and even where they are traced through or to any person whose parents are not or have not been married to one another. (2A)

Any step-parent or former step-parent who has sexual intercourse with his or her step-child or former step-child shall be guilty of an offence if that step-child is either under the age of twenty-one or has at any time before attaining the age of eighteen lived in the same household and been treated as a child of his or her family, unless the accused proves that he or she: did not know that this person was a step-child or former step-child; or, believed on reasonable grounds that s/he was of or over twenty-one years of age; or, did not consent to sexual intercourse with that person; or, was married to that person at the time sexual intercourse took place by a marriage entered into outside Scotland and recognised as valid by Scots law. (2B)

Any person of or over the age of sixteen years who has sexual intercourse with a child under the age of sixteen years and who is a member of the same household as that child and who is in a position of trust or authority in relation to that child shall be guilty of an offence unless s/he proves that s/he: believed on reasonable grounds that the person was of or over the age of sixteen years; or, did not consent to have sexual intercourse or to have sexual intercourse with that person; or, was married to that person at the time sexual intercourse took place by a marriage entered into outside Scotland and recognised as valid by Scots law. (2C)

On conviction on indictment in the High Court of Justiciary, a person found guilty is liable to imprisonment for any term up to and including life imprisonment. On conviction on indictment before the sheriff, a person found guilty is liable to imprisonment for a term not exceeding two years. On summary conviction, s/he is liable to imprisonment not exceeding three months. (2D, 5)

Before passing sentence on a person convicted of any such offence, the court shall a) obtain information about that person's circumstances from an officer of a local authority or otherwise and consider that information; and b) take into account any information before it which is relevant to his character and to his physical and mental condition. (2D, 6)

APPENDIX II
List of parliamentary debates

1903 Bill
>c. 1R Feb. 24 [118] 680
>2R Mar. 5 [118] 683
>Com. June 26 [124] 697
>3R June 26 [124] 706
>l. 1R June 29 [124] 724
>2R July 16 [125] 820
>Considered in Committee [H. C.], June 26 [124] 697

1908 Bill
>c. 1R Feb. 27 [185] 72
>2R Mar. 10 1436
>Report from Standing Committee Apr. 1 [187] 521
>3R July 3 1090
>l. 1R July 6 1149
>2R July 6 1149
>Com. and Rep. Dec. 3 1597
>c. Lords Amendts, Con. Dec. 16 1972
>l. Royal Assent Dec. 21 2346

1986 Bill
>c. 2R (16.05.86) 97 c1030
>Rep and 3R (4.07.86) 100 c1348–58
>Royal Assent (18.07.86) 101 c1367
>l. 1R [468] (21.11.85) 660
>2R and committed to a Ctte of the Whole House [469]
>   (9.12.85) 63–9
>Ctte [470] (28.1.86) 614–26
>Report [471] (24.2.86) 883
>3R and Passed [472] (11.3.86) 570
>Returned from the Commons Agreed to with Amendts [478]
>   (7.7.86) 158
>Commons Amendts considered (14.7.86) 737–8
>Royal Assent (18.7.86) 1085

NOTES

1 INTRODUCTION: INTERROGATING INCEST

1 I am thinking here of the work of Lévi-Strauss, Durkheim, Malinowski, amongst others. Even Freud, and later Parsons, who suggested that (unconscious) incestuous wishes were an important feature of normal psychological development, saw the incest prohibition as an unquestionable social fact, and Freud wrote an elaborate thesis on the origins of the incest prohibition.

2 I do not mean to suggest that there has never been any feminist interest in the incest prohibition. Gayle Rubin's influential article 'The Traffic in Women: Notes on the "Political Economy" of Sex' (1975) drew upon, *inter alia*, Lévi-Strauss' theory of exchange. Thus Rubin kept a central role for the incest prohibition in her theory, arguing that the exchange of women that the prohibition 'initiates' is central in the social relations of sex and gender.

3 This phrase was taken from a judge's summing up speech in a sexual abuse case in 1925. Jeffreys argues that the attitude it expresses has continued to the present time.

2 A CONTINUAL CONTEST: FOUCAULT AND FEMINISM

1 Reading Foucault in the early 1990s, one is struck by the further changes in sexual discourses. The way of speaking about sex which Foucault attacks, that which celebrates sexual liberation, has long since passed. Of course, Foucault's thesis concerning the historical and discursive production of sexuality is not contradicted by this.

2 A term adopted and adapted from Nietzche's (1968) 'will to power'.

3 The sense in which Foucault uses the term 'law' here is subject to debate (Cousins and Hussain, 1984: 236–8). Foucault seems to be using a very simple, stylised notion of law. It may be that he uses 'law' to refer not to the institution of law, which can use the other forms of power he discusses, but to a dominant image of law as an authority issuing commands.

4 Foucault used the term 'analytics' because he did not want to

construct a theory of power so much as a way of studying power's operations.

5 Foucault's war imagery is sometimes unhelpful to an understanding of his arguments because it carries with it notions that are not akin to his position, such as that of two sides in violent combat (Cousins and Hussain, 1984: 245–8).

6 Foucault's generalisation of disciplinary techniques to a notion of a 'disciplinary society' has been criticised as a move resembling the totalising notions of power which he opposed. The argument is more convincing when discussing the specific settings of disciplinary power without generalising its operations (Minson, 1985: 97–9; Breuer, 1989: 240–2).

7 Foucault (1980a: 146–7) argues that concern with centralised observation predated Bentham's Panopticon, but it was Bentham's 'device' which was repeatedly drawn upon in plans to recognise prisons from the first half of the nineteenth century.

8 It has also been used elsewhere in feminist work, such as in work on eating disorders (Bordo, 1990b).

9 This is not to say that Foucault cut off discourse from other non-discursive aspects of social life in *The Archaeology of Knowledge*. He has never divorced discourse from other factors that shape societies, such as economic ones. His point was to move away from the general division between discourse and the non-discursive world and to focus instead on a specific discourse – such as that on sexuality – in order to question the power relations within and outside the discourse, the knowledges it uses and instigates and its effects, including its effects on other discourses. However, in *The Archaeology of Knowledge* Foucault does seem to want to argue for or at least consider the autonomy of discourse in a way that he later does not (see Dreyfus and Rabinow, 1986: 67, 77–8).

10 Pierre Boncenne's (the interviewer's) words.

11 The archaeologist who 'diagnoses' discourses in relation to the broader 'reigning episteme' – the 'discursive regularities' and relations that unite sciences (1972: 191) – becomes the genealogist who begins from within them, reflecting on the world around him. Having begun in this way, the next manoeuvre is an archaeological one in which the genealogist 'can move one step back from the discourse he is studying and treat it as a discourse-object' (Dreyfus and Rabinow, 1986: 106). Thus genealogy still contains elements of archaeology within it (Dreyfus and Rabinow, 1986: 103–4).

12 Butler (1990b: 340) discusses how this assumption informs scientific works on sex determining genes, and cites Loewenstein (1987: 88–9).

13 Her reading is a generous one, for Foucault's position does not seem as persuasive or consistent as Butler presents it.

14 Thus Foucault's argument is not the classic relativist one that people's perceptions are always relative to their position in time and space (see Lukes and Hollis, 1982), but an argument about the relationship that can exist between power and the 'truths' that we accept and 'make function' as true.

15 This is the argument that Foucault had with 'rights talk'.

16 I use the term 'may' here because it is not the case that Foucault saw every form of knowledge and every knowledge claim as necessarily linked with power. He said that his claims were focused on the human sciences, for example, not on the 'exact' sciences (1988: 106).

17 However, this later clarification on his position reveals that Taylor's (1986) point was in part valid where he argued that the notion of power is linked *conceptually* with the notion of imposition so that Foucault's notion of power requires the notion of (what Taylor calls) freedom even if this possibility is empirically impossible.

3 FAMILIAR STORIES: THE FEMINIST ANALYSES OF INCEST

1 The fear of violence also means that women are constrained before any such incidents happen to them (Hanmer and Saunders, 1984).

2 Especially where it includes rape, which with babies and young children can be fatal (Rush, 1974, 1980; Ward, 1984: 141; Driver, 1989: 182). Driver lists some of the injuries that can follow child sexual abuse: lacerations, bleeding, bruises, grasp or bite marks; urinary tract infection, discharge, or venereal disease; the child may suffer anal dilation or dropped bowel, pain when urinating, vomiting, stomach ache, abdominal cramps. Then there are the psychosomatic symptoms of incontinence, eczema, asthma, allergies, nausea, fainting, and fits resembling epilepsy (1989: 182).

3 Where the capitalised form Father is used, I am, following Ward, referring not to biological fathers but to the role of an adult who would generally be expected to be caring and responsible toward the child. This may be the father, or the step-father, but the term is also used to include other relations and non-relations who are not strangers. Having said this, one should note that some of the arguments of this section apply with greater weight to a situation whereby the abuser lives in the same household as the abused. A similar implication is intended through the capitalisation of Mother, Daughter and Son. Ward also capitalises the Family to refer to an idealised and normalised institution.

4 When Foucault speaks about disciplinary power in *THS* he is speaking about the operations of power/knowledge in institutional settings and at work around the family (especially clear in the case of charitable institutions). Disciplinary power, as one pole of bio-power, operates 'around' the family, even as it draws lines within it: between parents and children, as one axis, and between the sexes, as another. Within a Foucauldian framework feminist concern about incest and the family would be seen to join with this biopolitical concern, encircling the family with 'pastoral agents'. Thus the feminist critique of the family no longer appears as a radical critique but as a mere continuation of one begun elsewhere by different groups and discourses. However, to adopt such a perspective would be to collapse feminist work into Foucault's scheme. If, on the other hand, we remain for the time being within the feminist discourse our

attention will be focused much more *'inside'* the family, discussing the dynamics of activity within it rather than around it. Of course feminists are aware that the operations of power within the family are influenced, constructed, directed even, by what occurs 'outside' the family; the family is always within an economic and cultural context. Nevertheless, the tendency of the feminist approach is to consider how power operates within the household setting. The feminist knowledge is based on the accounts given by survivors. Thus the point of entry is qualitatively different from Foucault's.

5 This argument may apply to boy children as much as to girl children, although the argument is insufficiently developed in feminist work to attribute this argument to any individual analysis.

6 By so labelling such states of domination Foucault seems to be reinstating exactly that form of power he had denied, but, as explained in Chapter 2, it is the distinction between structural power being always already there and it being built up through the tactics of power that he falls back on in this interview (1988: 19).

7 For example, some women may have authority in the home, and women teachers may have authority within a class, but this does not link them with a dominating group of people in a continuous state of domination.

8 A similar function is played by Hollway's use of Lacan. Although steeped in a different tradition, that of psychoanalysis, Lacan is introduced into the Foucauldian framework in order to describe the way in which discourses are incorporated into subjectivity.

9 Recent work on sexual abuse has revealed that many children who have been abused do tell somebody, but that they are either not heard at all, or are heard in such a way that the extent of sexual assault is not publicly known (Kelly *et al.*, 1991). This raises the question of conditions of hearing, something which Foucault, with his concentration on speaking, left unexplored.

10 Ward also looks at the myths as they surround the different actors: the Daughters, the Mothers, the Fathers. However, as I have suggested, her theoretical approach is somewhat different, since it is much more akin to an analysis of ideology, such as that of Althusser (1971).

11 For further discussion of feminist critique of family therapy see Goldner (1985), Hare-Mustin (1987) and Perelberg and Miller (1990).

12 I do not mean to imply a rigid distinction between 'feminists' and 'incest survivors' here. Some of the feminist works on incest are by women who have survived incestuous abuse, and of course many incest survivors are feminists.

13 As discussed above, the survivors are not untouched by the abusers' ways of 'explaining' the abuse.

4 TELLING AND TABOO: FEMINISM WITHIN THE FOUCAULDIAN LANDSCAPE

1 Foucault's arguments are not without their ambiguities, and any utilisation of them involves interpretation and elaboration.

2 Incidentally, there is a parallel problem with Foucault's writings on juridico-discursive power, in that Foucault never really clarifies whether this model of power actually existed in times past, or whether it is (merely) an historically recent way of speaking about an 'old' power.

3 The interviewing and work that has been done with incest abusers may be another matter.

4 This is of course almost exactly the line argued by Labour MP Stuart Bell in the 'Cleveland controversy' (see Campbell, 1988).

5 It is worth remembering that Foucault did not suggest that there has been a progression from one end (the kinship/blood end) to the other. Although incest prohibition is conservative in the sense that it tends to construct the family/kinship system both as functional and as desirable, it is articulated simultaneously with those discourses which focus on the incest act. Both exist contemporaneously. Neither are the latter straightforwardly more 'progressive'. Although they recognise the occurrence of incest, these ways of talking can enter power networks, for example, by regarding offenders as sexually perverted in a way that avoids questioning the exercise of power within the family.

6 This argument is reminiscent of that of Miller (1990), who suggests that when the rhetoric of the harmonious family is threatened by a violent act, family members will reinterpret the violent member as in some sense 'outside' the family, declaring 'he's not the man I married', 'he's no son of mine', etc. (1990: 275).

7 One might add that the work of other authors on the incest prohibition have seen it as productive. For example, Lévi-Strauss saw the incest prohibition as productive. For him, it resulted in exogamy which produced social interdependence and culture itself.

8 Lindzey also argues that incestuous desire would be the least remarkable of sexual attractions given the fact that people tend to choose people like themselves and family members would presumably share the most in common, a good example of incest being set up as an omnipresent danger in the family at the same time as the existence of a strong incest prohibition is upheld.

9 I am referring here to my arguments on power in Chapter 3 where it was argued that power is not a possession, but that its exercise can be perpetually asymmetrical and that the family is probably the prime example where although power is negotiated it remains almost 'perpetually asymmetrical' along lines of both gender and age.

5 WHAT'S THE PROBLEM? THE CONSTRUCTION AND CRIMINALISATION OF INCEST

1 Except for the period 1650–61 when the Puritan Commonwealth made incest punishable by death. Apparently, however, the 1650 Act was largely a 'dead letter' (Bailey and Blackburn, 1979).

2 Although the 1857 Matrimonial Causes Act did specify 'incestuous adultery' as grounds for divorce.

3 The details of the Acts are contained in Appendix I; the list of parliamentary debates is contained in Appendix II.

4 Subjects which have been debated by scholars with regard to the English legislation. See Bailey and Blackburn (1979), Wolfram (1983), Jeffreys (1985).

5 I do not make any arguments about individuals' consistency; one speaker may draw upon several different knowledges. Nor, since my purpose is not to present a history of change in the legal discourse on incest, shall I attempt to make generalisations about changes over time between the two periods. The purpose is to investigate how the debates that shaped the current legislation in English and Scots law constructed incest as a problem.

6 See also the Under Secretary of State for the Home Department, Herbert Samuel, 26.6.1908, Commons, and the Lord Chancellor, Lord Loreburn, 2.12.1908, Lords.

7 The others are: maintaining the solidarity of the family; prevention of psychological harm to family members; and the opinion that society as a whole would wish incest to remain criminal.

8 This question is left unanswered.

9 This phrase is used to separate these constructions of the wrong of incest from those that see incest as wrong because of the effects upon future generations or upon an abstract institution such as the family.

10 Bill 51. Later, son was added to the female's list of criminalised relationships.

11 Here the SLC draw on the work of Benward and Densen-Gerber (1975).

12 The Law Commission had initially recommended against this inclusion (in the Memorandum), but were persuaded otherwise by the commentators on that Memorandum, and the recommendation for inclusion is made in the Report.

13 This point, whilst drawing on Foucault, also echoes the criticism of him for implicitly mapping repressive 'old' modes of power on to law. Law does not operate in a contrary fashion to bio-power, but is itself the site of the operations of power/knowledge.

14 For further discussion of how this perspective differs from other feminist analyses of law, see Naffine (1990).

6 MAKING MONSTERS, LOCATING SEX: FOUCAULT AND FEMINISM IN DEBATE

1 Both debates are translated and reprinted in Foucault (1988).

2 See p. 15–18 above.

3 There has been much debate around the phrase Foucault uses toward the end of *THS*: 'The rallying point for the counterattack against the effects of the deployment of sexuality ought not to be sex-desire, but bodies and pleasures (1981: 157). Some critics have argued that this was an appeal to something 'fundamental' under the effects of the deployment of sexuality. I think it was not an appeal to an essential and unchanging experience so much as a

suggestion that we rethink the language we use, to subvert current ways of understanding desire.

4 Foucault also seems to be making a further suggestion: that rape might become a civil rather than a criminal offence, so that instead of criminal prosecution of the perpetrator, women would claim compensation after having been raped. In this discussion, however, I will consider only his first suggestion, that of punishing rape as a physical and not a sexual assault.

5 Marine Zecca is introduced as 'collaborator of David Cooper', who is a doctor and psychiatrist.

6 Foucault does not really make it clear why we would *want* to challenge the deployment in all its manifestations.

7 It should be noted that Plaza takes Foucault to be advocating the legal desexualisation of rape whereas in my reading it remains ambiguous as to whether he is actually recommending the change or just simply presenting the question as a dilemma for his theoretical point of view. For the purposes of this chapter, however, it will be supposed that Foucault did give weight to 'desexualisation' as a political strategy.

7 CONCLUSION

1 As I have mentioned above, there are various terms used to describe the location of incest as a form of sexual violence. There has been some debate within feminism that suggested that 'incest' was in danger of losing its specificity in feminist parlance as the term 'child sexual abuse' gained currency. At one time there was furthermore a supposition that all child sexual abuse was incestuous (Kelly, 1988a). The two terms are presently in use within feminist discussions as linked issues but with certain specificities.

2 For discussion of the sexual abuse of boys see, e.g., Bolton *et al.* (1989).

3 And, less obviously perhaps, vice versa.

4 Such as the Sachs and Wilson (1978) study, or the very different work of MacKinnon (e.g. 1983).

5 Foucault's work has been used in feminist analyses of law before, by Edwards (1981). However, Edwards' work uses Foucault, amongst others, to investigate the one area of 'female sexuality' as it is drawn into the legal sphere (e.g. in rape trials). Smart's work, on the other hand, uses Foucault in a much broader way, building suggestions for the study of all law from a feminist perspective. For this reason I concentrate upon Smart's analyses.

6 A phrase from Virginia Woolf's *A Room of One's Own* (1973). Cline and Spender (1988) suggest that reflecting men at twice their natural size is an unreciprocated task that women carry out for men.

BIBLIOGRAPHY

Adams, M.S. and Neal, J.V. (1967) 'Children of Incest', *Pediatrics* 40.

Adams, P. (1979) 'A Note on Sexual Division and Sexual Difference', *m/f: A Feminist Journal* 3.

Adler, Z. (1987) *Rape on Trial*, Routledge & Kegan Paul: London.

Alcoff, L. (1988) 'Cultural Feminism versus Post-Structuralism: The Identity Crisis in Feminist Theory', *Signs: A Journal of Women in Culture and Society* 13: 3.

Althusser (1971) 'Ideology and Ideological State Apparatuses (Notes Toward an Investigation)', in *Lenin and Philosophy*, Monthly Review Press: New York.

Amir, M. (1971) *Patterns in Forcible Rape*, University of Chicago Press: Chicago.

Arens, W. (1986) *The Original Sin: Incest and Its Meaning*, Oxford University Press: New York.

Armstrong, L. (1978) *Kiss Daddy Goodnight: A Speak Out On Incest*, Hawthorn Books, Inc.: New York.

Armstrong, L. (1987) *Kiss Daddy Goodnight: Ten Years Later*, Pocket Books: New York.

Atkins, S. and Hoggett, B. (1984) *Women and the Law*, Basil Blackwell: Oxford.

Badgley, R., Allard, H., MaCormick, N., Proudfoot, P., Fortin, D., Oglivies, D., Re-Grant, Q., Celinas, P., Pepin, L.and Sutherland, S. (Committee on Sexual Offences Against Children and Youth) (1984) *Sexual Offences against Children* (Vol. 1), Canadian Government Publishing Centre: Ottawa.

Bailey, V. and Blackburn, S. (1979) 'The Punishment of Incest Act 1908: A Case Study in Law Creation', *Criminal Law Review*, p. 708.

Baker, A. and Duncan, S. (1985) 'Child Sexual Abuse: A Study of Prevalence in Great Britain', *Child Abuse and Neglect* 9: 4.

Balbus, I. (1982) 'Disciplining Women: Michel Foucault and the Power of Feminist Discourse', *Praxis International* 5: 4.

Barale, M. (1986) 'Body Politics/Body Pleasured: Feminism's Theories of Sexuality, A Review Essay', *Frontiers: A Journal of Women's Studies* IX: 1.

Barbaree, H.E. and Marshall, W.L. (1989) 'Erectile Responses among Heterosexual Child Molesters, Father–Daughter Incest Offenders,

and Matched Non-offenders: Five Distinct Age Preference Profiles',
Canadian Journal of Behavioural Science 21: 1.

Barrett, M. and McIntosh, M. (1982) *The Anti-Social Family*, NLB: London.

Barry, K. (1985) 'Social Etiology of Crimes Against Women', *Victimology* 10.

Bartkowski, F. (1988) 'Epistemic Drift in Foucault', in I. Diamond and L. Quinby (eds) *Feminism and Foucault: Reflections on Resistance*, Boston: Northeastern University Press.

Bartky, S. (1988) 'Foucault, Feminism and the Modernisation of Patriarchal Power', in I. Diamond and L. Quinby (eds) *Feminism and Foucault: Reflections On Resistance*, Boston: Northeastern University Press.

Becker, H. (1963) *Outsiders: Studies in the Sociology of Deviance*, Free Press of Glencoe: London.

Bell, V. (1991) 'Beyond the "Thorny Question": Feminism, Foucault and the Desexualisation of Rape', *International Journal of the Sociology of Law* 19: 1.

Bender, L. and Blau, A. (1937) 'The Reactions of Children to Sexual Relations with Adults', *American Journal of Orthopsychiatry* 7.

Benward and Densen-Gerber (1975) 'Incest as a Causative Factor in Anti-Social Behaviour: An Exploratory Study', *Contemporary Drug Problems* 4.

Bernauer, J. and Rasmussen, D. (eds) (1988) *The Final Foucault*, MIT Press: Cambridge, Mass.

Bolton, F., Morris, L. and MacEachron, A. (1989) *Males at Risk: The Other Side of Child Sexual Abuse*, Sage: London.

Bordo, S. (1990a) 'Feminism, Postmodernism and Gender Scepticism', in L. Nicholson (ed.) *Feminsm/Postmodernism*, Routledge: New York.

Bordo, S. (1990b) 'Reading The Slender Body', in M. Jacobus, E. Keller and S. Shuttleworth (eds) *Body/Politics: Women and the Discourses of Science*, Routledge: New York.

Braidotti, R. (1991) *Patterns of Dissonance: A Study of Women in Contemporary Philosophy*, Basil Blackwell: Oxford.

Breuer, S. (1989) 'Foucault and Beyond: Towards a Theory of the Disciplinary Society'. *International Social Science Journal* 41: 2.

Brownmiller, S. (1975) *Against Our Will: Men, Women and Rape*, Secker & Warburg: London.

Burman, M. (1989) 'Constructing Consent: Statutory Sexual Offences and the "Rape-Model" ', Paper presented at the British Criminology Conference, Bristol.

Butler, J. (1990a) *Gender Trouble: Feminism and the Subversion of Identity*, Routledge: New York.

Butler, J. (1990b) 'Gender Trouble: Feminist Theory and Psychoanalytic Discourse', in L. Nicholson (ed.) *Feminism/Postmodernism*, Routledge: New York.

Butler, S. (1985) *Conspiracy of Silence: The Trauma of Incest*, Volcano Press, Inc: San Francisco. (First published 1978.)

Cameron, D. and Fraser, E. (1987) *The Lust to Kill*, Polity Press: Cambridge.

Campbell, B. (1988) *Unofficial Secrets: Child Sexual Abuse – The Cleveland Case*, Virago Press: London.

Chodorow, N. (1979) *The Reproduction of Mothering: Psychoanalysis and the Sociology of Gender*, University of California Press: London.

Cline, S. and Spender, D. (1988) *Reflecting Men: At Twice Their Natural Size*, Fontana: London.

Cohen, S. and Scull, A. (1985) *Social Control and the State: Historical and Comparative Essays*, Basil Blackwell: Oxford.

Connell, N. and Wilson, C. (eds) (1974) *Rape: The First Sourcebook for Women*, New American Library: New York.

Cousins, M. and Hussain, A. (1984) *Michel Foucault*, Macmillan: Basingstoke.

Daly, M. (1978) *Gyn/Ecology*, Women's Press: London.

De Lauretis, T. (1987) *Technologies of Gender*, Macmillan: Basingstoke.

Diamond, I. and Quinby, L. (eds) (1988) *Feminism and Foucault: Reflections on Resistance*, Northeastern University Press: Boston.

Dominelli, L. (1986) 'Father–Daughter Incest', *Critical Social Policy* 16.

Dominelli, L. (1989) 'Betrayal of Trust: A Feminist Analysis of Power Relationships in Incest Abuse and Its Relevance for Social Work Practice', *British Journal of Social Work* 19.

Donzelot, J. (1979) *The Policing of Families* (trans. by R. Hurley), Hutchinson: London.

Dreyfus, H. and Rabinow, P. (1986) *Michel Foucault: Beyond Structuralism and Hermeneutics*, Harvester Press: Brighton. (First published 1982, University of Chicago Press: Chicago.)

Driver, E. (1989) 'Introduction', in E. Driver and A. Droisen (eds) *Child Sexual Abuse: Feminist Perspectives*, Macmillan: Basingstoke.

Droisen, A. (1989) 'Some Autobiographies', in E. Driver and A. Droisen (eds) *Child Sexual Abuse: Feminist Perspectives*, Macmillan: Basingstoke.

Dumaresq, D. (1981) 'Rape – Sexuality in the Law', *m/f: A Feminist Journal* 5/6.

Durkheim, É. (1963) *Incest: The Nature and Origin of the Taboo*, Lyle Stuart: New York. (First published in French, 1898, trans. E. Sagarin.)

Dworkin, A. (1981) *Pornography: Men Possessing Women*, The Women's Press: London.

Edwards, A. (1987) 'Male Violence in Feminist Theory: An Analysis of the Changing Conceptions of Sex/Gender Violence and Male Dominance', in J. Hanmer and M. Maynard (eds) *Women, Violence and Social Control*, Macmillan: Basingstoke.

Edwards, S. (1981) *Female Sexuality and the Law*, Martin Robertson: Oxford.

Ember, M. (1983) 'On the Origin and Extension of the Incest Taboo', in M. Ember and C.R. Ember (eds) *Marriage, Family and Kinship: Comparative Studies of Social Organisation*, Human Relations Area Files Press: Newhaven, Conneticut.

Feminist Review (1988) *Family Secrets: Child Sexual Abuse*, Special Issue, 28, Spring.

Finkelhor, D. (1984) *Child Sexual Abuse: New Theory and Research*, Free Press: New York.

Finkelhor, D., Hotaling, G., Lewis, I.A. and Smith, C. (1990) 'Sexual Abuse in a National Survey of Adult Men and Women: Prevalence, Characteristics and Risk Factors', *Child Abuse and Neglect* 14.

Foucault, M. (1970) *The Order of Things*, Tavistock: London. (First published in French, 1966.)

Foucault, M. (1972) *The Archaeology of Knowledge* (trans. A.M. Sheridan-Smith), Tavistock: London. (First published in French, 1969.)

Foucault, M. (1977) *Language, Counter-Memory, Practice: Selected Essays and Interviews* (ed. by D. Bouchard; trans. by D. Bouchard and S. Simon), Cornell University Press: Ithaca, NY.

Foucault, M. (1979a) *Discipline and Punish* (trans. by A.M. Sheridan-Smith), Penguin: London (First published in French, 1975. This translation first published 1977, Allen Lane: London.)

Foucault, M. (1979b) *Power, Truth, Strategy* (ed. M. Morris and P. Patton), Feral Publications: Sydney.

Foucault, M. (1980a) *Power/Knowledge: Selected Writings 1972–1977* (ed. by C. Gordon; trans. by C. Gordon, L. Marshall, J. Meplam and K. Soper), Harvester Press: Brighton.

Foucault, M. (1980b) 'Introduction' to *Herculine Barbin: Being the Recently Discovered Memoirs of A Nineteenth-Century French Hermaphrodite* (trans. by R. McDougall), Harvester Press: Brighton. (First published in French, 1973.)

Foucault, M. (1981) *The History of Sexuality Volume 1: An Introduction* (trans. by R. Hurley), Penguin: Harmondsworth. (First published in French, 1976. This translation first published 1979, Allen Lane: London.)

Foucault, M. (1986a) *The Foucault Reader* (ed. by P. Rabinow), Penguin: Harmondsworth.

Foucault, M. (1986b) 'The Subject and Power' (trans. L. Sawyer), Afterword in N. Dreyfus and P. Rabinow, *Michel Foucault: Beyond Structuralism and Hermeneutics*, Harvester Press: Brighton. (First published 1982, University of Chicago Press: Chicago.)

Foucault, M. (1988) *Politics, Philosophy, Culture: Interviews and Other Writings 1977–1984* (ed. by L. Kritzman), Routledge: New York.

Fraser, N. (1981) 'Foucault on Modern Power: Empirical Insights and Normative Confusions', *Praxis International* 1.

Fraser, N. (1985) 'Michel Foucault: A Young Conservative?', *Ethics* 96.

Fraser, N. (1989) *Unruly Practices: Power, Discourse and Gender in Contemporary Social Theory*, Polity Press: Cambridge.

Freud, S. (1977) *Three Essays on Sexuality* (trans. J. Strachey), Penguin: Harmondsworth. (First published in German, 1905.)

Freud, S. (1983) *Totem and Taboo* (trans. J. Strachey), Routledge & Kegan Paul: London. (First published in German, 1913.)

Freud, S. and Breuer, J. (1956) *Studies on Hysteria* (trans. J. and A. Strachey), Hogarth Press: London. (First published in German, 1895.)

Gebhard, P., Gagnon, J., Pomeroy, W. and Christenson, C. (1965) *Sex Offenders: An Analysis of Types*, Harper & Row: New York.

Goldner, V. (1985) 'Feminism and Family Therapy', *Family Process* 24.

Goodrich, P. (1987) *Legal Discourse*, Macmillan: Basingstoke.

Goody, J. (1971) 'Incest and Adultery', in J. Goody (ed.) *Kinship: Selected Readings*, Penguin: Harmondsworth.

Gordon, L. (1986) 'Incest and Resistance: Patterns of Father–Daughter Incest', *Social Problems* 33: 4.

Gordon, L. (1988) *Heroes of Their Own Lives: The Politics and History of Family Violence*, Viking: New York.

Griffin, S. (1982) 'The Politics of Rape', in *Made From This Earth: Selections From Her Writing 1967–82*, Women's Press: London. (First published 1971 as 'Rape – The All-American Crime'.)

Gunew, S. (1990) 'Feminist Knowledge: Critique and Construct', in S. Gunew (ed.) *Feminist Knowledge: Critique and Construct*, Routledge: London.

Hacking, I. (1986) 'The Archaeology of Foucault', in D. Hoy (ed.) *Foucault: A Critical Reader*, Basil Blackwell: Oxford.

Hacking, I. (1991) 'The Making and Molding of Child Abuse', *Critical Inquiry* 17, Winter.

Hanmer, J. and Saunders, S. (1984) *A Well-Founded Fear: A Community Study of Violence to Women*, Hutchinson: London.

Harding, S. (1987) 'The Instability of the Analytical Categories of Feminist Theory', in S. Harding and J. O'Barr (eds) *Sex and Scientific Inquiry*, University of Chicago Press: Chicago. (First published 1986 in *Signs: A Journal of Women in Culture and Society* 11: 4.)

Hare-Mustin, R. (1987) 'The Problem of Gender in Family Therapy Theory', *Family Process* 26.

Hartmann, H. (1981) 'The Unhappy Marriage of Marxism and Feminism: Towards a More Progressive Union', in L. Sargent (ed.) *Women and Revolution*, Pluto Press: London.

Hartsock, N. (1990) 'Foucault on Power: A Theory for Women?', in L. Nicholson (ed.) *Feminism/Postmodernism*, Routledge: New York.

Hawkeshead, M. (1989) 'Knowers, Knowing, Known: Feminist Theory and Claims of Truth', *Signs: A Journal Of Women in Culture and Society* 14: 3.

Hekman, S. (1990) *Gender and Knowledge: Elements of a Postmodern Feminism*, Polity Press: Cambridge.

Henriques, J., Hollway, W., Urwin, C., Venn, C. and Walkerdine, V. (1984) *Changing the Subject: Psychology, Social Regulation and Subjectivity*, Methuen: London.

Herman, J. and Hirschman, L. (1977) 'Father–Daughter Incest', *Signs: A Journal of Women in Culture and Society* 2: 3.

Herman, J. with Hirschman, L. (1981) *Father–Daughter Incest*, Harvard University Press: Cambridge, Mass.

Hollway, W. (1984) 'Gender Difference and the Production of Subjectivity', in Henriques, J., Hollway, W., Urwin, C., Venn, C. and Walkerdine, V. *Changing the Subject: Psychology, Social Regulation and Subjectivity*, Methuen: London.

Hudson, D. (1987) 'You Can't Commit Violence against An Object: Women Psychiatry and Psychosurgery', in J. Hanmer and M. Maynard (eds) *Women, Violence and Social Control*, Macmillan: Basingstoke.

Huth, A.H. (1875) *The Marriage of Near Kin Considered with Respect to the Law of Nations, the Results of Experience and the Teachings of Biology*, Longmans, Green & Co.: London.

Irigaray, L. (1985) *Speculum of the Other Woman* (trans. by G. Gill), Cornell University Press: Ithaca, NY. (First published in French, 1974.)

Jackson, S. (1978) *On the Social Construction of Female Sexuality* (Explorations in Feminism No. 4), Women's Research and Resources Centre Publication: London.

Jeffreys, S. (1982) 'The Sexual Abuse of Children in the Home', in S. Friedman and E. Sarah (eds) *On the Problem of Men*, Women's Press: London.

Jeffreys, S. (1985) *The Spinster and Her Enemies: Feminism and Sexuality 1880–1930*, Pandora: London.

Justice, B. and Justice, R. (1979) *The Broken Taboo: Sex in the Family*, Peter Owen: London.

Kaplan, G. and Rogers, L. (1990) 'The Definition of Male and Female: Biological Reductionism and the Sanctions of Normality', in S. Gunew (ed.) *Feminist Knowledge: Critique and Construct*, Routledge: London.

Kaufman, I., Peck, A. and Tagiuri, C. (1954) 'The Family Constellation and Overt Incestuous Relations between Father and Daughter', *American Journal of Orthopsychiatry* 24.

Kelly, L. (1988a) 'What's in a Name?', Special Issue, *Feminist Review* 28, Spring.

Kelly, L. (1988b) *Surviving Sexual Violence*, Sage: London.

Kelly, L., Regan, L. and Burton, S. (1991) 'An Exploratory Study of the Prevalence of Sexual Abuse in a Sample of 16–21 Year Olds', Polytechnic of North London.

Kempe, R. and Kempe, C.H. (1978) *Child Abuse*, Open Books: London.

Kitzinger, C. (1987) *The Social Construction of Lesbianism*, Sage: London.

Kitzinger, J. (1988) 'Defending Innocence: Ideologies of Innocence', Special Issue, *Feminist Review* 28, Spring.

La Fontaine, J. (1990) *Child Sexual Abuse*, Polity Press: Cambridge.

Lees, S. (1986) *Losing Out: Sexuality and Adolescent Girls*, Hutchinson: London.

Lemert, C. and Gillan, G. (1982) *Michel Foucault: Social Theory and Transgression*, Columbia University Press: New York.

Lévi-Strauss, C. (1969) *The Elementary Structures Of Kinship* (translated by J. Bell, and J. Von Sturmer, with R. Needham), Eyre & Spottiswoode: London. (First published in French, 1949.)

Liddle, M. (1989) 'Feminist Contributions to an Understanding of Violence against Women – Three Steps Forward, Two Steps Back', *Canadian Review of Sociology and Anthropology* 26: 5.

Lindzey, G. (1967) 'Some Remarks Concerning Incest, the Incest Taboo and Psychoanalytic Theory', *American Psychologist* 22.

Loewenstein, J. (1987) 'The Conundrum of Gender Identification: Two Sexes are Not Enough', *Pacific Discovery* 40: 2.

Lukes, S. (1986) *Power*, New York University Press: New York.

Lukes, S. and Hollis, M. (eds) (1982) *Rationality and Relativism*, Basil Blackwell: Oxford.

Lukianowicz, N. (1972) 'Incest', *British Journal of Psychiatry* 120.

Lyotard, F. (1984) *The Postmodern Condition: A Report on Knowledge* (trans. by G. Bennington and B. Massumi), Manchester University Press: Manchester. (First published in French, 1979).

MacKinnon, C. (1982) 'Feminism, Marxism, Method and the State: An Agenda for Theory', *Signs: A Journal of Women in Culture and Society* 7: 3.

MacKinnon, C. (1983) 'Feminism, Marxism, Method and the State: Toward Feminist Jurisprudence', *Signs: A Journal of Women in Culture and Society* 8: 4.

MacKinnon, C. (1987) *Feminism Unmodified: Discourses on Life and Law*, Harvard University Press: Cambridge, Mass.
MacKinnon, C. (1989) *Toward a Feminist Theory of the State*, Harvard University Press: Cambridge, Mass.
MacLeod, M. and Saraga, E. (1988) 'Challenging the Orthodoxy', Special Issue, *Feminist Review* 28, Spring.
McNeill, S. (1987) 'Flashing: Its Effect on Women', in J. Hanmer and M. Maynard (eds), *Women, Violence and Social Control*, Macmillan: Basingstoke.
McWhorter, D. (1986) 'Theory and Beyond: Foucault's Relevance for Feminist Thinking', Unpublished PhD, Vanderbilt University.
Maisch, H. (1972) *Incest*, Stein & Day: New York.
Malinowski, B. (1927) *Sex and Repression in a Savage Society*, Routledge & Kegan Paul: London.
Marcuse, H. (1956) *Eros and Civilisation: A Philosophical Enquiry into Freud*, Routledge & Kegan Paul: London.
Martin, B. (1988) 'Feminism, Criticism and Foucault', in I. Diamond and L. Quinby (eds) *Feminism and Foucault: Reflections on Resistance*, Northeastern University Press: Boston.
Mason, J.K. (1981) '1567 and All That', *The Scots Law Times*, 18 December.
Masson, J. (1985) *The Assault on Truth: Freud's Suppression of the Seduction Theory*, Penguin: Harmondsworth. (Originally published 1984, Farrar, Strauss & Giroux: New York.)
Mauss, M. (1970) *The Gift: Forms and Functions of Exchange in Archaic Societies* (trans. by I. Cunnison), Routledge & Kegan Paul: London. (First published in French, 1925.)
Medea, A. and Thompson, K. (1974) *Against Rape*, Farrar, Strauss & Giroux: New York.
Melani, L. and Fodaski, L. (1974) 'The Psychology of the Rapist and his Victim', in N. Connell and C. Wilson (eds) *Rape: The First Sourcebook for Women*, New American Library: New York.
Merquoir, J. (1985) *Foucault*, Fontana: London.
Miller, A. (1985) *Thou Shalt Not Be Aware: Society's Betrayal of the Child*, Pluto Press: London.
Miller, L. (1990) 'Violent Families and the Rhetoric of Harmony', *British Journal of Sociology* 41: 2.
Minson, J. (1981) 'The Assertion of Homosexuality', *m/f: A Feminist Journal* 5/6.
Minson, J. (1985) *Genealogies of Morals: Nietzsche, Foucault, Donzelot and the Eccentricity of Ethics*, Macmillan: Basingstoke.
Morris, M. (1988) *The Pirate's Fiancée: Feminism, Reading, Postmodernism*, Verso: London.
Naffine, N. (1990) *Law and the Sexes*, Allen & Unwin: London.
Nelson, S. (1982) *Incest: Fact and Myth*, Stramullion: Edinburgh.
Neu, J. (1985) 'What is Wrong with Incest?', in R. Wasserstrom (ed.) *Today's Moral Problems*, Macmillan: Basingstoke.
Nietzsche, F. (1968) *The Will to Power* (trans. by W. Kaufmann), Vintage: New York.

O'Donnell, C. and Craney, J. (1982) *Family Violence in Australia*, Longman Cheshire: Melbourne.

Parsons, T. (1954) 'The Incest Taboo in Relation to Social Structure and the Socialisation of the Child', *British Journal of Sociology* 5.

Pateman, C. (1988) *The Sexual Contract*, Polity Press: Cambridge.

Perelberg, R.J. and Miller, A.C. (1990) *Gender and Power in Families*, Routledge: London.

Peterson, S. (1977) 'Coercion and Rape: The State as a Male Protection Racket', in M. Vetterling-Braggin, F. Elliston and J. English (eds) *Feminism and Philosophy*, Littlefield: Totowa, NJ.

Phelan, S. (1990) 'Foucault and Feminism', *American Journal of Political Science* 34: 2.

Plaza, M. (1980) 'Our Costs and Their Benefits' (trans. by W. Harrison) *m/f: A Feminist Journal* 4.

Potter, J. and Wetherell, M. (1987) *Discourse and Social Psychology: Beyond Attitudes and Behaviour*, London: Sage.

Rajchman, J. (1985) *Michel Foucault: The Freedom of Philosophy*, Columbia University Press: New York.

Reich, W. (1975) *The Invasion of Compulsory Sexual Morality*, Penguin: Harmondsworth. (First published in German, 1932. This translation originally published 1971 Farrar, Straus & Giroux: New York.)

Rich, A. (1980) 'Compulsory Heterosexuality and Lesbian Existence', in C. Stimpson and E. Person (eds) *Women: Sex and Sexuality*, Chicago University Press: Chicago.

Rubin, G. (1975) 'The Traffic in Women: Notes on the "Political Economy" of Sex', in R. Reiter (ed.) *Toward an Anthropology of Women*, Monthly Review Press: New York.

Rubin, G. (1984) 'Thinking Sex: Notes For a Radical Theory of the Politics of Sexuality', in C. Vance (ed.) *Pleasure and Danger: Exploring Women's Sexuality*, Routledge & Kegan Paul: London.

Rush, F. (1974) 'The Sexual Abuse of Children: A Feminist Point of View', in N. Cornell and C. Wilson (eds) *Rape: The First Sourcebook for Women*, New American Library: New York.

Rush, F. (1980) *The Best Kept Secret: Sexual Abuse of Children*, McGraw-Hill Book Company: New York.

Russell, D. (1975) *The Politics of Rape*, Stein & Day: New York.

Russell, D. (1984) *Sexual Exploitation: Rape, Child Sexual Abuse and Workplace Harassment*, Sage: Beverly Hills.

Russell, D. (1986) *The Secret Trauma: Incest in the Lives of Girls*, Sage: Beverly Hills.

Sachs, A. and Wilson, J. (1978) *Sexism and the Law: A Study of Male Beliefs and Judicial Bias*, Martin Robertson: Oxford.

Sawicki, J. (1988) 'Feminism and the Power of Foucauldian Discourse', in J. Arac (ed.) *After Foucault: Humanistic Knowledge, Postmodern Challenges*, Rutgers University Press: New Brunswick.

Sawicki, J. (1991) *Disciplining Foucault: Feminism, Power and the Body*, Routledge: New York.

Schor, N. (1987) 'Dreaming Dissymmetry: Barthes, Foucault and Sexual

Difference', in A. Jardine and P. Smith (eds) *Men in Feminism*, Methuen: New York.

Scottish Law Commission (1980) *The Law of Incest in Scotland*, Memorandum No. 44.

Scottish Law Commission (1981) *The Law of Incest in Scotland: Report on a Reference under Section 3 (1) (e) of the Law Commissions Act 1965*, Cmnd 8422, Her Majesty's Stationery Office: Edinburgh.

Seemanova, E. (1971) 'A Study of Children of Incestuous Mating', *Human Heredity* 21.

Segal, L. (1992) 'Sensual Uncertainty, Or Why the Clitoris is Not Enough', in H. Crowley and S. Himmelweit (eds) *Knowing Women: Feminism and Knowledge*, Polity/OUP: Cambridge.

Shulman, A. (1980) 'Sex and Power: Sexual Bases of Radical Feminism', in C. Stimpson and E. Person (eds) *Women: Sex and Sexuality*, Chicago University Press: Chicago.

Smart, C. (1984) *The Ties That Bind: Law, Marriage and the Reproduction of Patriarchal Relations*, Routledge & Kegan Paul: London.

Smart, C. (1989) *Feminism and the Power of Law*, Routledge: London.

Smart, C. (1990) 'Feminist Approaches to Criminology, or Postmodern Woman Meets Atavistic Man', in L. Gelsthorpe and A. Morris (eds) *Feminist Perspectives in Criminology*, Open University Press: Milton Keynes.

Snitow, A., Stansell, C. and Thompson, S. (1984) *Desire: The Politics of Sexuality*, Virago Press: London.

Stanko, E. (1985) *Intimate Intrusions: Women's Experience of Male Violence*, Routledge: London.

Stern, L. (1980) 'Introduction to Plaza', *m/f: A Feminist Journal* 4.

Taylor, P. (1986) 'Foucault on Freedom and Truth', in D. Hoy (ed.) *Foucault: A Critical Reader*, Basil Blackwell: Oxford.

Temkin, J. (1986) 'Women, Rape and Law Reform', in R. Porter and S. Tomascelli (eds) *Rape*, Basil Blackwell: Oxford.

Turkel, G. (1990) 'Michel Foucault: Law, Power and Knowledge', *Journal of Law and Society* 17: 3.

Vance, C. (1984) (ed.) *Pleasure and Danger: Exploring Female Sexuality*, Routledge & Kegan Paul: London.

Vance, C. (1992) 'Social Construction Theory: Problems in the History of Sexuality', in H. Crowley and S. Himmelweit (eds) *Knowing Women: Feminism and Knowledge*, Polity/OUP: Cambridge.

Vega, J. (1988) 'Coercion and Consent: Classic Liberal Concepts in Texts on Sexual Violence', *International Journal of the Sociology of Law* 16.

Vicinus, M. (1982) 'Sexuality and Power: A Review of Current Work in the History of Sexuality', *Feminist Studies* 8: 1.

Walby, S. (1986) *Patriarchy at Work: Patriarchal and Capitalist Relations in Employment*, Polity Press: Cambridge.

Waldby, C., Clancy, A., Emetchi, J. and Summerfield, C. (1989) 'Theoretical Perspectives on Father–Daughter Incest', in E. Driver and A. Droisen (eds) *Child Sexual Abuse: Feminist Perspectives*, Macmillan: Basingstoke.

Wapner, P. (1989) 'What's Left?: Marx, Foucault and Contemporary Problems of Social Change', *Praxis International* 9: 1/2.

Ward, E. (1984) *Father–Daughter Rape*, Women's Press: London.

Wasoff, F. (1980) 'What is Wrong with Incest?', *SCOLAG*.

Watney, S. (1986) 'The Banality of Gender', *Oxford Literary Review* 8: 1.

West, R. (1989) 'Feminism, Critical Social Theory and Law', University of Chicago Legal Forum.

Westermarck, E. (1921) *The History of Human Marriage*, Macmillan: London. (First published 1894.)

Wilson, E. (1983) *What is to be Done about Violence Against Women?*, Harmondsworth: Penguin.

Wolfram, S. (1983) 'Eugenics and the Punishment of Incest Act 1908', *Criminal Law Review*, p. 308.

Woodhull, W. (1988) 'Sexuality, Power and the Question of Rape', in I. Diamond and L. Quinby (eds) *Feminism and Foucault: Reflections on Resistance*, Northeastern University Press: Boston.

Woolf, V. (1973) *A Room of One's Own*, Penguin: Harmondsworth. (First published 1928.)

Young, F. (1967) 'Incest Taboos and Social Solidarity', *The American Journal of Sociology* 72: 6.

INDEX

adultery 143
affinity, decriminalising of
    intercourse between relations
    by 142, 144
Althusser, L. 74
archaeology 42–5, 167
Armstrong, L. 64, 69, 78, 109
authority, power as 60–2, 72

Barbin, H. 50–1
Bartky, S. 37–8, 69
Becker, H. 8
body, the 19, 32, 33–4, 37–9,
    50–1, 64, 68, 70, 159, 161–3,
    164–5, 168, 171–2
boys, abuse of 102, 176
Brownmiller, S. 102, 155, 176
Butler, J. 50–3, 114–16
Butler, S. 65, 79

Cameron, D. 76, 122, 124
Chesler, P. 78
children: adopted 142; and
    adult–child sex (debate)
    151–60; and court procedures
    175, 183–4; definition of 147,
    151; and familial power
    relations 66–7; girl-children as
    seductive 85–7; of incest
    130–2, 134, 144; and
    incestuous desires 120; and
    innocence 86; and obedience
    60–1; in object relations
    theory 110–12; neglected
    137–8; responsibility of

mother for 83–4, 107–8; and
    sexuality 17, 18, 36, 77–9, 81,
    86, 94, 96, 99, 151–60, 172;
    step-children 127, 132, 136,
    139, 143, 145, 147; 'training'
    of girl-children 67–9; as
    unheard 104
Chodorow, N. 110
Cohen, S. 7–9
confession 19–20, 46–7, 101–4
consciousness-raising 49
consent vii, viii, 10, 122, 127,
    132–3, 139, 143, 146–7,
    151–2, 155–9, 160, 166–7,
    172, 183–4
continuum, of male violence 58
Cousins, M. 16–17

Danet, J. 151, 152, 157
De Lauretis, T. 68, 74, 75, 163
decriminalisation: of adult–child
    sex 151–60; of sexual relations
    between relations of affinity
    142, 144
desexualisation 161–2, 164–5
deployment of alliance 93–100,
    143, 146
disciplinary power see power
discourse: analysing legal 127–9;
    Foucault on 42–7; Foucault
    and feminism on 47–56,
    79–91; see also
    power/knowledge; subjugated
    knowledges; truth
domination see power

207